# The Radiology Survival Guide

# The Radiology Survival Guide

## Dr Chris Cook

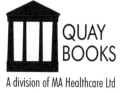

QUAY
BOOKS

A division of MA Healthcare Ltd

Quay Books Division, MA Healthcare Ltd, St Jude's Church, Dulwich Road, London
SE24 0PB

British Library Cataloguing-in-Publication Data
A catalogue record is available for this book

© MA Healthcare Limited 2007

ISBN-13: 978 1 85642 314 4
ISBN-10: 1–85642–314–X

Printed in the UK by Athenaeum Press Ltd, Dukesway, Team Valley, Gateshead, NE11 0PZ

# Contents

# Acknowledgements

I would like to thank the following for their help in providing some of the images/cases used in this book; Drs S Barnard, J Brown, T Campbell-Smith, C Costello, R Hopkins, G Stoddart, C Styles.

I would also like to thank my family for their support in writing this book, and to J Anderson, M Hampshire, O Hickey, T Parsons (of Medical Illustration, Bristol Royal Infirmary), and all at Quay Books for their professional help.

I would like to dedicate this book to my parents.

# Introduction

The aim of this book is systematically to review examples of the radiological appearances of commonly encountered pathologies. It is designed to be used not only as a reference text but also as a 'self-test' book.

The *Radiology Survival Guide* is written primarily to be of interest to medical students, F1 and F2 year postgraduate doctors (formerly the house officer and senior house officer years of training). However, due to the depth of information given, it is also anticipated to be of use in the preparation for postgraduate examinations including MRCP and MRCS.

In essence, this text should prove invaluable for the medical student prior to the sitting of final examinations, and provides 'all you need to know' for the day-to-day work of the junior doctor.

The *Radiology Survival Guide* is divided into seven sections:

- the chest radiograph
- the abdominal radiograph
- musculoskeletal radiology
- intravenous urography and imaging of the urinary tract.
- ultrasound, computed tomography, and magnetic resonance imaging
- computed tomography of the brain
- interventional radiology

Each section begins with an introduction to the basics of radiological interpretation, and includes 'key points' which act as a part summary. This is followed by a series of cases within each section that provide a pictorial summary of the commonly encountered pathologies. Each case begins with a radiograph and radiological 'report', and this is then followed by relevant background material.

This book is written in an easy to understand style, and clinical information is also given where relevant. The section on computed tomography of the brain has been included due to the likelihood of these examinations being provisionally reported by non-radiological staff in the near future. The section on interventional radiology has been included due to the author's realisation of the need for more awareness of this sub-speciality among junior medical staff, and the increasing reliance on minimally invasive procedures within modern medical practice.

# Section 1

## The Chest Radiograph

## Introduction

The chest radiograph (or chest X-ray, CXR) is one of the most widely requested radiographic examinations but is also one of the most difficult to evaluate accurately. A basic scheme for CXR evaluation is invaluable and should include all the points covered below.

### Patient details

Patient details are annotated on the radiograph at the time of its being taken. The patient's age and name, and possibly the geographical position of the hospital may all give important clues as to subsequent pathology, whether it be sex preponderance in certain malignancies, or inhalational exposure-related diseases in known industrial areas.

### Radiographic analysis

Consider the following:

* postero-anterior (PA) or antero-posterior (AP) projection
* exposure
* rotation
* the side marker.

The *standard projection* in which chest X-rays are taken in an X-ray department is the *PA projection*. This is sometimes annotated on the radiograph, but this projection is so much the norm that if there is no such marking it is usually safe to assume that the radiograph has been taken in this way. By comparison, if the radiograph has been taken AP, this is invariably marked as such on the film, either by a subtle 'AP' next to the patient details, or it is written elsewhere on the film by the radiographer at the time of the exposure. AP films are usually taken if the patient is too ill for the PA projection, for example in cases of trauma, or in mobile (ie. non-departmental) chest radiographs.

The radiograph *exposure* is both subjective and objective. Historically, the correct exposure should just allow visualisation of the vertebral end-plates through the mediastinum.

*Rotation* can be assessed by overall symmetry of the thoracic cavity, and in particular by ensuring that the distance from the spinous process (a posterior structure) with the medial end of the clavicles (anterior structures) are the same on both sides. If this distance is decreased, this suggests that the patient is rotated forward on that side (see *Figure 1A*).

It is important to ensure that the *side marker* is present and in the expected position; remember, however, that it is more likely for the radiographer to have placed the side marker incorrectly than for the patient to be suffering from dextrocardia!

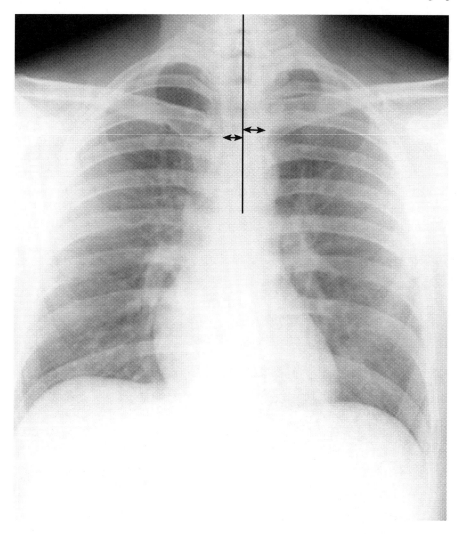

*Figure I A. CXR with a line drawn along the spinous processes, and measured from the medial end of both clavicles. Note the decreased distance on the left side indicating the patient is rotated with the left side of the chest rotated anteriorly; ie. a left anterior oblique rotation.*

### Patient factors

The following factors should be considered:

* expansion/inspiratory effort
* medical supportive/monitoring equipment, eg. ECG electrodes, endotracheal tube.

Patients are asked to breath in prior to taking a chest X-ray. The *inspiratory effort* made by the patient is assessed by counting the number of ribs seen above the level of the hemidiaphragms. Anteriorly, it is usual to be able to see 6 or 7 costochondral cartilage joints, while posteriorly, 9 or 10 ribs are usually seen (*Figure 1B*). The flatness of the hemidiaphragms is also useful in assessing the degree of inspiratory effort.

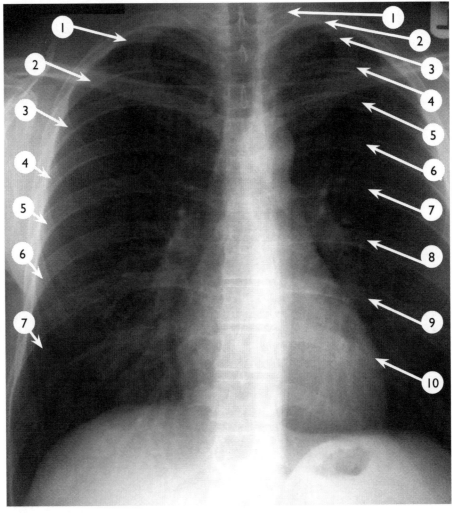

*Figure 1B. CXR showing numbered ribs (anterior, right ribs; posterior, left ribs). Note the normal superimposition of the posterior ribs at the lung apex.*

The extent to which a patient has made inspiratory effort depends on both pathological and non-pathological factors. Over-inspiration may be seen in otherwise young and fit individuals, but may also be seen in asthmatics or in those suffering from chronic obstructive pulmonary disease (COPD). Under-expansion may be seen in people with poor motivation, or with obesity, or in the elderly, as well as in a generally sick patient or a patient with restrictive (fibrotic) lung disease.

The documentation of wires or other *medical supportive or invasive equipment*, may be useful in giving clues as to the patient's overall clinical state. In addition, these features should be reviewed when evaluating the radiograph to ensure that they are all suitably positioned, and that no complications from their insertion have occurred. For example, an endotracheal tube should be positioned in the mid trachea, and certainly at least 1 or 2 cm above the carina. Central venous catheters ('central lines') placed within the great vessels should have their tips within the superior vena cava, or within the right atrium, and complicating pneumo- or haemothoraces should be excluded. A tube inserted for drainage of pleural fluid should usually be positioned with its tip directed inferiorly towards the lung base, and pneumothorax secondary to its insertion should be excluded.

Although all of the above are important in preliminary chest X-ray analysis, the heart/mediastinum and lungs are now considered in detail.

### Heart and mediastinum

Here we will look at:

* mediastinal contours
* heart shape and size, including the cardiothoracic ratio (CTR).

The mediastinum includes the following structures: the heart, central pulmonary vessels, aorta, trachea and oesophagus. These may be seen outlined on the chest radiograph in *Figure 1C*.

Although some authorities suggest that the mediastinum is widened on the PA CXR when measured at more than 8 cm in transverse diameter at the level of the carina, most radiologists' opinions of the mediastinal contours and size are subjective.

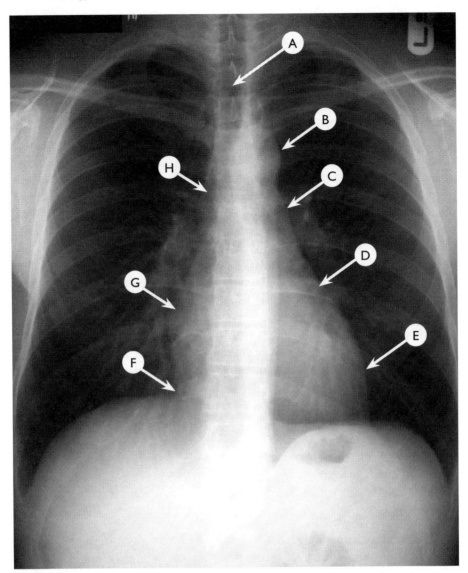

*Figure I C. CXR with heart and mediastinal structures labelled A to H. Note that the oesophagus is not usually seen unless distended and gas filled. A, trachea; B, aortic knuckle; C, pulmonary artery; D, left atrial appendage; E, left ventricle; F, inferior vena cava; G, right atrium; H, superior vena cava.*

Artefactual widening of the mediastinum is common. This occurs because the mediastinal structures are positioned anteriorly, and are therefore magnified on AP films, especially when taken supine. As such, the mediastinum often appears widened or equivocal on the supine AP film but is shown to be normal on a subsequent erect PA radiograph. An erect PA CXR should therefore be obtained whenever possible.

The causes of true mediastinal widening can be divided into *vascular* and *non-vascular*. Vascular causes of mediastinal widening can be differentiated from non-vascular causes such as lymph node enlargement by the recognition of a smooth vascular contour and the continuation of this contour with known vascular structures such as the aorta or the subclavian arteries.

The *cardiothoracic ratio* (CTR) is a measurement of *heart size*. The CTR (in adults normally less than 50%) is assessed by the ratio of the widest breadth of the heart to the widest internal diameter of the thoracic cavity (see *Figure 1D*). These measurements are made in centimetres, and the CTR is stated as (for example) '15 on 34'. The CTR will thus be increased in conditions such as cardiac failure, but equally may be decreased if there is relative over-expansion of the lung fields, as may occur in COPD.

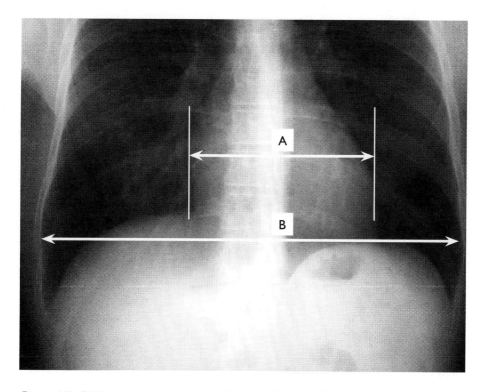

*Figure 1D. CXR with maximum heart (A) and thoracic (B) diameters annotated on the radiograph. The CTR is defined as the ratio of distance A to distance B.*

The hila represent the positions of entry of the pulmonary vessels and airways into the lungs, but on the chest radiograph they are largely seen as a result of the pulmonary vessels. The right hilum is normally positioned at a level slightly higher than its left-sided counterpart. The hila should be of similar density on both sides; beware of the unilateral dense hilum which may be due to a subtle hilar mass due to bronchogenic carcinoma.

Hilar enlargement occurs either due to hilar lymphadenopathy (secondary to a variety of different pathologies, as listed below) or due to enlargement of the pulmonary vessels if there is increased flow through them. This may occur in response to hypoxaemia secondary to diffuse pulmonary disease. This 'secondary pulmonary hypertension' is most usually seen in cases of COPD. Alternatively, pulmonary artery enlargement may more rarely be seen secondary to increased blood flow from the right side of the heart; due, for example, to left-to-right shunts as a result of atrial or ventricular wall defects. Rarely, pulmonary hypertension occurs as a primary entity.

Causes of bilateral hilar enlargement include:

- Vascular
    - pulmonary hypertension
- Hilar lymphadenopathy
    - sarcoidosis
    - lymphoma
    - atypical infections (eg. viral, histoplasmosis).

Causes of unilateral hilar enlargement are usually due to lymphadenopathy (although pulmonary artery aneurysm does rarely occur):

- lymph nodes secondary to lung malignancy (look for an associated mass)
- lymphoma
- infective (eg. tuberculosis).

### Lung fields

The normal lung parenchyma contains both vascular and bronchial structures. However, the vascular structures are more apparent on the plain chest radiograph. These vessels originate at the hila, and are composed of both pulmonary arteries and veins (supplying and draining the blood for oxygenation) and bronchial arteries and veins (supplying the needs of the lung parenchyma itself).

Abnormal lung markings may be categorised thus:

* nodules or masses
* interstitial (and/or reticular) markings
* air-space changes.

*Masses* (greater than 1 cm in diameter) are usually readily detected by virtue of their size. Conversely, *nodules* (less than 1 cm in diameter) can be extremely difficult to see, and may be either obscured by or confused with the adjacent vascular markings. A good test of the true presence of a nodule is the 'tweezer test' (whether one can imagine actually picking it out of the adjacent lung parencyhma with tweezers). In doing this it soon becomes clear that it is genuinely particulate, and is not continuous with nearby vessels, or other linear markings.

*Interstitial markings* are linear markings (lines) that cannot be attributed to normal lung markings. These are usually less than 1 mm in thickness and are of variable length (usually 2–3 cm). A good example of this can be seen in *Case 1.10*. The description of a *reticular pattern* means purely 'net-like'. A reticular pattern may occur due to a certain density of interstitial markings whereby overlapping lines eventually give the appearances of a net. A reticular–nodular pattern may occur due to a combination of linear and nodular appearances, but is more likely to occur due to the eye perceiving nodules within the reticular pattern at the point of the interstitial lines overlapping. It is therefore a term which is probably best avoided.

*Air-space changes* occur due to the air within normally aerated lung being replaced by fluid or cellular infiltrate. Fluid may take the form of *pus* (in cases of pneumonia), *transudate* or *exudate* (in cases of cardiac, renal or hepatic failure, etc), *blood* (due to trauma), or more rarely *cellular infiltrate* (alveolar cell carcinoma).

Causes of air-space opacification are therefore summarised as:

* pus (pneumonia)
* blood (trauma, pulmonary haemorrhage)
* transudate/exudate (cardiac, renal or hepatic failure)
* cellular infiltrate (alveolar cell carcinoma).

Air-space changes are classically poorly defined (easily remembered as 'cloud-like') and if persistent aeration is present within the bronchi, then these air-filled tubular structures may be seen as they pass through the area of consolidation. This is called an 'air bronchogram' (*Figure 1E*).

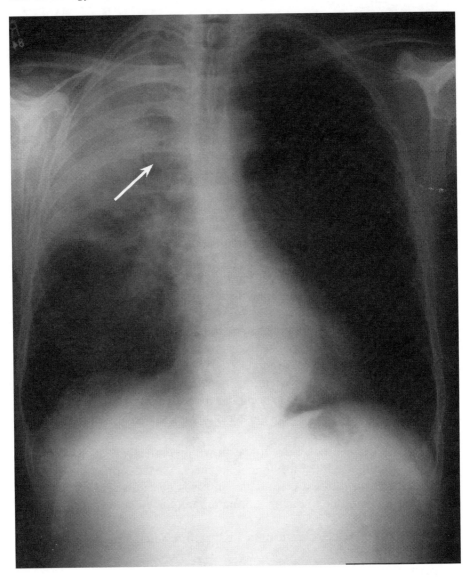

*Figure I E. CXR showing collapse and consolidation of the right upper lobe. Note the low density of air still seen within the segmental bronchi (arrow).*

From the preceding discussion it is apparent that there is a wide differential diagnosis of air-space opacification. The cause of air-space opacification on any one film may be clarified by other contributory findings on the radiograph. For example, air-space changes due to cardiac failure will usually be bilateral and symmetrical and there may be associated cardiomegaly, pleural effusion or upper lobe venous distension. Pneumonia will usually be seen within a single localised area and an air bronchogram may be present. Clinical correlation is also important as with all radiograph interpretation.

### Pleural surfaces (including diaphragms)

The pleura surrounds the lung and both hemidiaphragms and is not usually seen. It may however be thickened or calcified. The diaphragms are normally dome-like structures, with the right being slightly higher then its left counter-part due to the liver beneath. There may sometimes be several curves to each diaphragm (known as eventration) although their presence is of no signifi-cance. The diaphragms can become flattened in cases of hyperexpansion, for example in COPD (see *Case 1.16*), and calcification may also be seen from previous TB (*Figure 1.4b*) or asbestos exposure (*Case 1.5*). Most importantly, free gas beneath the diaphragm must be excluded, since this indicates intra-abdominal perforation. This must not be confused with the normal stomach gas bubble (see *Figure 1.14c*).

### Review areas

These are areas of the radiograph that should be routinely evaluated since pathology is easily obscured by normal anatomical outlines or is visually less apparent. In medical student examinations, or for the MRCP, these areas should be remembered if the initial radiograph evaluation has not revealed any obvious pathology.

The review areas are as follows:

- *Behind the heart*: mass lesions or left lower lobe collapse and consolidation can easily be obscured by the cardiac silhouette.
- *Lung apices*: numerous overlying ribs may obscure subtle pathology.
- *Sub-diaphragmatic*: remember to look for free gas or intra-abdominal mass lesions.
- *Bones*: as a rule, inexperienced observers concentrate on the mediastinum and lung fields, and often fail to see either evidence of diffuse bone abnormality (eg. prostatic metastases as in *Case 3.2*) or focal bone lesions (eg. subtle areas of bone lysis or sclerosis).
- *Soft tissues on the edge of film*: these areas are often not evaluated by inexperienced observers.

**Key points of chest radiology**

Remember the importance of a scheme for CXR analysis. This is summarised below:

- Patient details.
- Radiographic analysis.
- Patient factors.
- Heart and mediastinum (anatomical contours, CTR, etc.).
- Lung fields (nodule/mass, interstitial markings, air-space changes).
- Pleural surfaces and diaphragms.
- Review areas.

## CASE 1.1 Aortic aneurysm

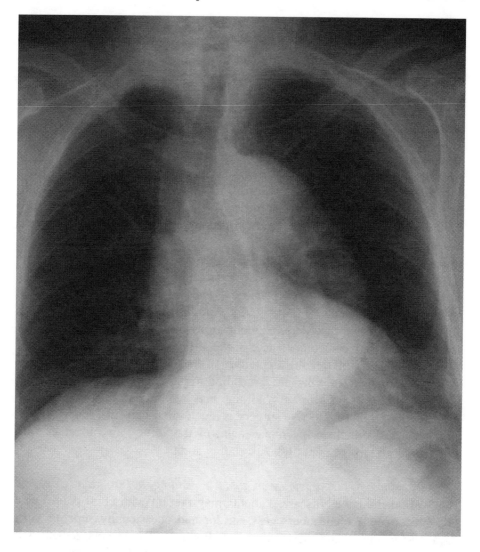

There is widening of the mediastinum with a smooth outline suggesting this is likely to be due to a vascular cause such as aortic aneurysm. There is no evidence of haemothorax, and thus no radiological evidence of rupture on plain film, although CT may be indicated to further evaluate the aortic calibre and extent of the aneurysm involvement into the descending aorta and abdomen. In cases of aortic rupture, CT will also demonstrate the presence of mediastinal haematoma or haemothorax (blood in the pleural space).

## Background

Aneurysms may be true or false. True aortic aneurysms involve dilation of all three layers of the aortic wall, whereas false aneurysms (which are usually the result of contained ruptures) are contained only by the outer layer of the aorta (adventitia), with surrounding fibrosis and organised haematoma. Aneurysms of the thoracic aorta may include the ascending aorta, the arch or the descending aorta, either individually or in combination. Common aetiologies include atherosclerosis and connective tissue diseases. Aneurysm can be confused with aortic ectasia (unfolding), although the aortic diameter should not be dilated in the latter.

*Aneurysms of the ascending aorta* usually begin at the aortic root. Plain chest radiograph findings of an ascending aortic aneurysm include prominence of the right mediastinal border and cardiac enlargement if the left ventricle dilates as a consequence of aortic valve incompetence. Most cases are idiopathic, although Marfan and Ehler–Danlos syndromes do predispose. Syphilis was once a common cause of ascending aortic aneurysms but is now uncommon in developed countries. The aortic wall is often calcified in syphilitic aneurysms (*Figure 1.1a*). Similar appearances may be seen in connective tissue disorders. Complications of thoracic aortic aneurysms include aortic valve incompetence, aortic dissection and rupture. Medical treatment consists of treating hypertension and other risk factors. Surgery is often recommended when the ascending aortic diameter reaches 55 mm, although patients with Marfan syndrome may require earlier surgery due to higher risk of rupture. Elective surgery is much safer than emergency surgery and will usually include the replacement of the aortic valve together with synthetic graft replacement of the ascending aorta.

*Aneurysms of the aortic arch and descending aorta* are usually the result of atheromatous disease. Patients may present with chest pain. Local pressure effects include hoarseness, stridor and occasionally superior vena cava obstruction. Plain chest radiograph findings include enlargement and tortuosity of the aortic outline. Contrast-enhanced helical CT scanning is the preferred method of investigation (*Figure 1.1b*). Surgery for descending aortic aneurysms carries a higher risk of complications (especially paraplegia due to the interruptions of spinal arteries) and so the threshold for surgery is higher.

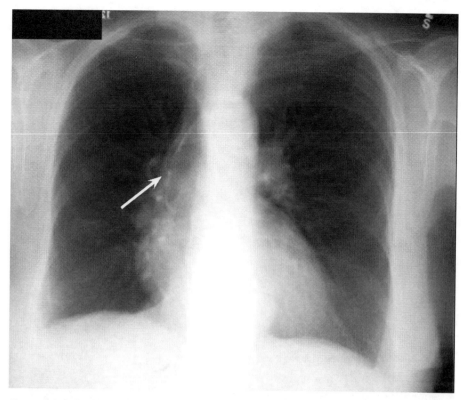

Figure 1.1a Classical ascending aortic aneurysm, with calcified wall in keeping with syphilitic aortitis (arrow).

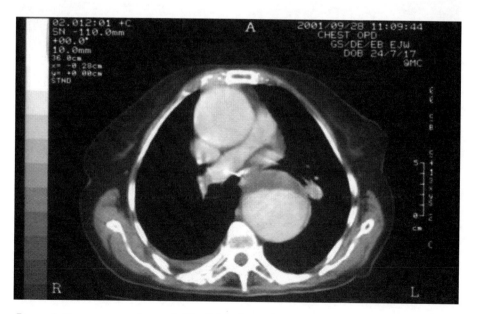

Figure 1.1b contrast-enhanced CT of the chest showing aneurysmal dilation of the ascending and descending aorta.

## CASE1.2 Sarcoid

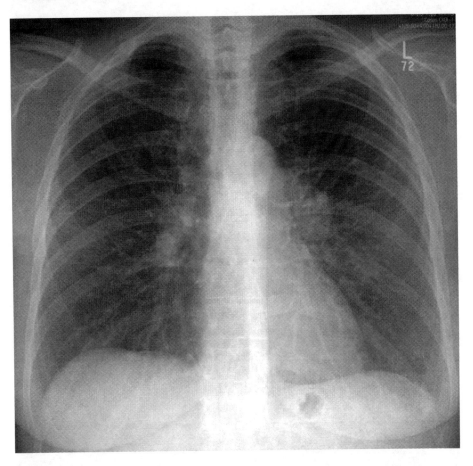

There is classical bilateral hilar lymphadenopathy. The appearances are those of sarcoidosis.

## Background

Sarcoid is a multisystem non-caseating granulomatous disorder that can involve almost any body system. It is most commonly seen within the respiratory and gastrointestinal tracts as well as the central nervous system. It also has important ocular manifestations including uveitis. Sarcoid gives a great variety of CXR appearances, ranging from the classical bilateral hilar lymphadenopathy as seen here, to upper-zone fibrotic change (*Figure 1.2a*), or multiple pulmonary nodules. In approximately 5% of cases, fine rims of calcific density are seen to surround the lymph nodes at both hila; so-called eggshell calcification (*Figure 1.2b*). These appearances can also occur in silicosis (see below).

Hilar nodes can be distinguished from mediastinal nodes by the lucent line that separates them medially from the mediastinum. The majority of patients with sarcoid will also have enlarged right paratracheal, aortopulmonary and subcarinal lymph nodes.

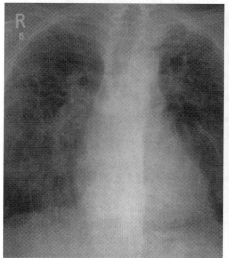

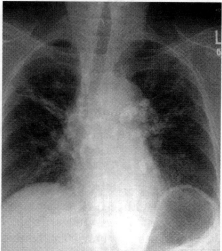

Figure 1.2a CXR showing linear changes in upper lobes due to fibrosis. Note that both hila are lying in elevated positions due to traction.

Figure 1.2b CXR showing eggshell calcification at both hila. There is also evidence of upper zone linear change in keeping with fibrosis. This is particularly prominent on the right side.

## Silicosis

This occurs due to long-term exposure to stone dust, and is thus an occupational exposure disease seen in quarry workers. The condition can give the same upper-zone fibrotic change and peripheral eggshell calcification of mediastinal lymph nodes that occurs in sarcoid. It can also result in widespread dense nodular change. An occupational history is essential.

## CASE 1.3 Multiple calcified nodules

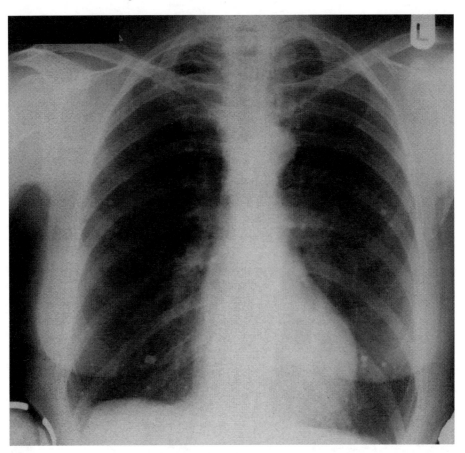

There are multiple nodules throughout both lung fields. They are 2–3 mm in diameter, and are of the same density as bone; and are thus calcified. The heart and mediastinum appear normal. These are the appearances of previous varicella pneumonia, and they are probably an incidental finding.

## Background

There is a differential diagnosis for the appearance of multiple calcified nodules. Common causes are:

* tuberculosis
* sarcoid
* silicosis
* mitral valve disease
* previous varicella pneumonia (chicken pox progressing to give viral pneumonia).

It may be difficult to differentiate sarcoid and silicosis without an occupational history. Tuberculosis may also give identical appearances, although pleural thickening and cavitation may be seen. Mitral valve disease may of course have other manifestations of cardiac disease such as cardiomegaly, left atrial enlargement, or other appearances due to cardiac failure. Calcified nodules due to previous varicella pneumonia are of 1–3 mm diameter, and occur in 2% of cases several years after the acute infection has resolved. They are usually an incidental finding.

## CASE 1.4 Tuberculosis

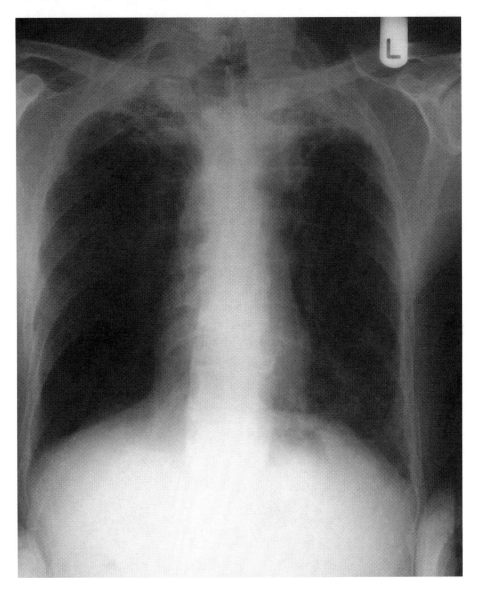

There is evidence of upper lobe fibrosis and cavitation in keeping with old tuberculosis. There is marked elevation of both hila and the trachea is significantly deviated to the right side due to a fibrotic reaction.

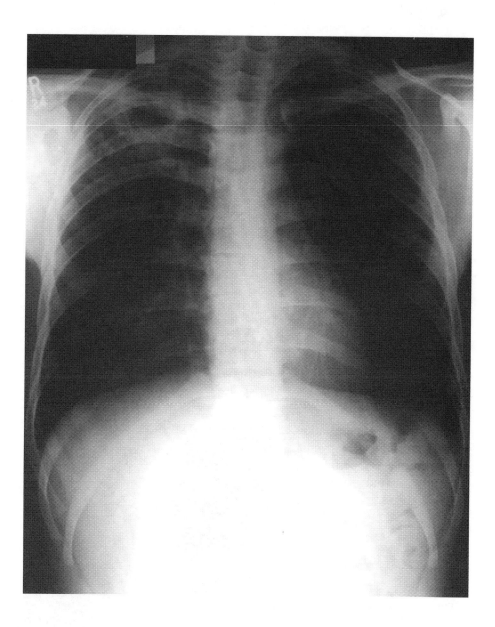

This image shows an extensive area of air-space opacification in the right upper lobe with associated cavitation. This patient recently resettled in the UK from central Asia. There is no significant hilar lymphadenopathy. The appearances are those of acute post-primary tuberculosis.

## Background

Primary tuberculosis (TB) is characterised by a small area of peripheral consolidation (*Figure 1.4a*) (Ghon focus) and hilar lymphadenopathy which can later calcify.

The classical appearance of active post-primary TB is of irregular, patchy consolidation in the apical bronchopulmonary segments of either lung (as in *Figure 1.4a*). These areas may subsequently cavitate, and healing occurs with fibrosis.

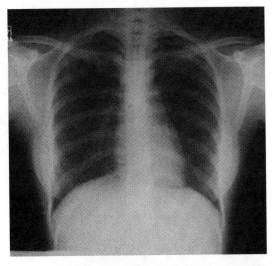

*Case 1.4a. CXR with poorly defined air-space opacification in keeping with active primary TB.*

An alternative manifestation is of tuberculous empyema which appears as a peripheral, pleurally based area of amorphous calcification (see *Figure 1.4b*). These appearances may resemble those changes seen after asbestos exposure, but they are unilateral, and of course occur in the absence of other features of asbestos-related lung disease.

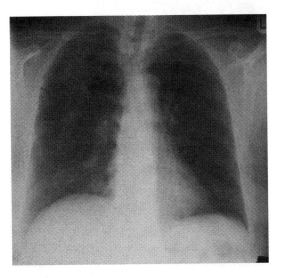

*Figure 1.4b. CXR with unilateral area of pleural calcification in typical 'holly leaf' configuration due to old TB empyema.*

Other features of TB exposure include the historical surgical manifestations:

- *Thoracoplasty*: rib resection to cause lung collapse (*Figure 1.4c*).
- *Plombage*: the insertion of foreign material (similar to ping-pong balls) to compress the adjacent infected lung.
- *Phrenic nerve crush*: to result in diaphragmatic elevation, and underinflation.

These were performed in order to collapse the infected segments, in the hope that this would prevent further spread, and aid healing. They are no longer performed, but may occasionally be seen in elderly patients.

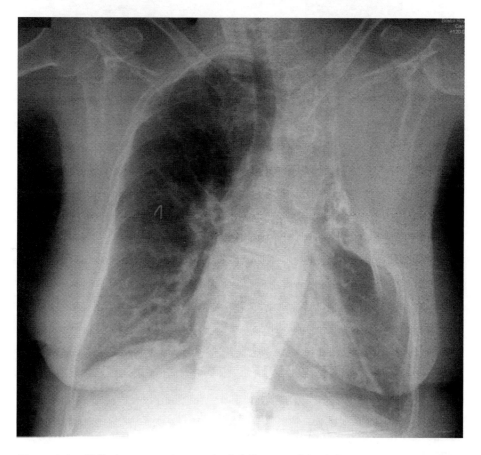

Figure 1.4c. CXR demonstrating marked deformity of the left upper chest wall due to multiple rib excisions. This is due to the historical operation known as thoraco-plasty. The metal clip in the right mid zone is artefactual.

## CASE 1.5 Asbestos-related lung disease

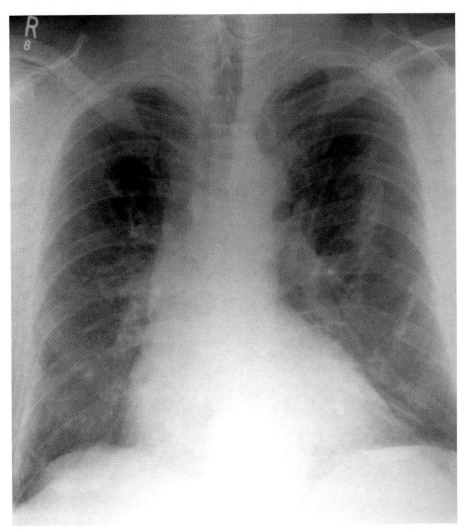

There is evidence of bilateral pleural thickening, and calcified pleural plaque giving a typical 'holly leaf' configuration. There is also subtle calcification of the left hemidiaphragm. These are the appearances of previous asbestos exposure.

## Background

Exposure to asbestos may give rise to a number of manifestations. These include pleural plaques, diffuse pleural thickening, pleural effusions and malignant mesothelioma.

Pleural plaques tend to calcify and are said to be 'holly leaf' in outline when seen *en face*. Plaques usually occur in the mid zones or overlying the hemidiaphragms and are often seen bilaterally (cf. the unilateral appearances of longstanding tuberculous empyema of old haemothorax). These changes may be associated with fibrotic interstitial lung disease (ie. asbestosis), which may be seen as basal linear interstitial markings on the plain chest radiograph, but is more accurately diagnosed using high-resolution (narrow section) CT of the chest.

## CASE 1.6 Lymphoma

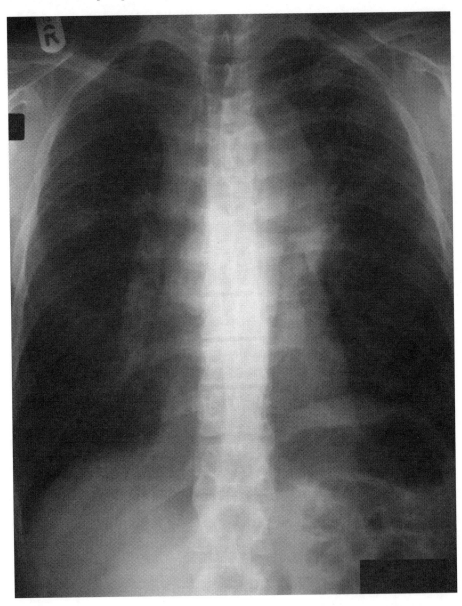

There is marked widening of the superior mediastinum, and both hila are enlarged in a symmetrical fashion. The lungs are clear, and the trachea appears central and of normal calibre. There is a differential for these appearances, but the most likely diagnosis is of lymphoma.

### Background

Lymphoma and leukaemia commonly cause anterior and paratracheal lymphadenopathy. The lymphadenopathy is usually bilateral but may be asymmetrical. Hodgkin's lymphoma more commonly causes lymph node enlargement than non-Hodgkin's lymphoma. The lymph node enlargement tends to surround adjacent organs, rather than invade them, and thus the trachea is less likely to be compressed in lymphoma than it is in cases of thyroid goitre or other mediastinal malignancies. These appearances of lymphadenopathy due to lymphoma can resolve rapidly after treatment.

Causes of mediastinal widening are:

* lymphoma
* goitre (thyroid enlargement)
* thymus enlargement (especially in infants)
* thymoma
* other rare tumours including teratoma.

*Thyroid enlargement (goitre)* is seen as a soft tissue density extending from the lower neck, occasionally resulting in a widened superior mediastinum. There may be evidence of tracheal shift or narrowing (see *Case 1.7*). The *thymus gland* usually lies anterior to the ascending aorta. It is large in neonates and infants, but atrophies with age and is not usually visible on the plain chest radiograph beyond childhood (see also p. 29). *Thymomas* are smooth in outline and are usually seen adjacent to the thoracic aorta (see also p. 29).

## CASE 1.7 Thyroid enlargement (goitre)

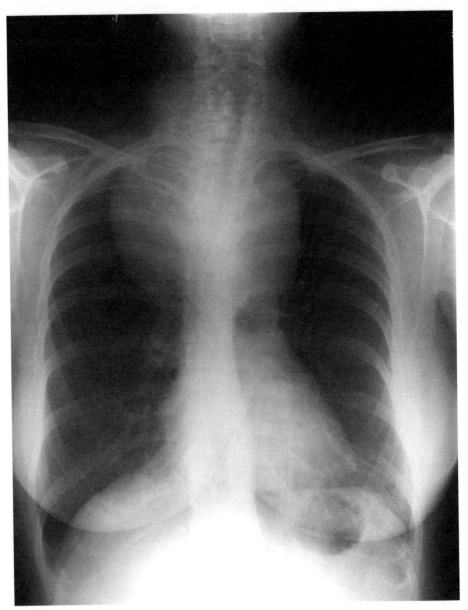

There is massive enlargement of the superior mediastinum extending into the neck. The trachea is deviated and appears narrowed. The appearances are in keeping with thyroid enlargement (goitre).

## Background

Thyroid enlargement (goitre) is often asymmetrical and can cause focal deviation and narrowing of the trachea. Goitre may extend down into the mediastinum from the neck. If a plain radiograph has indicated likely thyroid enlargement, then it is usually appropriate to further evaluate this by ultrasound which will indicate whether the enlargement is due to glandular tissue, cyst formation, or a more sinister focal mass which is more likely to represent primary thyroid malignancy. CT of goitre will show a well-defined soft tissue density in the paratracheal or retrotracheal region which is continuous with the thyroid tissue in the neck. Thyroid tissue is of higher attenuation than muscle on both unenhanced and enhanced scans due to the high iodine content of the normal gland. Thyroid enlargement is usually due to multinodular colloid goitre but occasionally adenoma or carcinoma can exist in an enlarged thyroid extending into the thorax. It is not possible to diagnose malignancy in the thyroid on CT unless there is local infiltrative spread beyond the gland.

Although lymphoma and goitre are the most common causes of mediastinal widening (see also *Case 1.6*) thymus gland enlargement and thymomas should be considered.

The *thymus gland* usually lies anterior to the ascending aorta. It is large in neonates and infants, but atrophies with age and should not be visible on the plain chest radiograph beyond childhood. Enlargement of the thymus may be due to thymoma, lymphoma, and other rare tumours.

*Thymomas* are smooth in outline. They may be large and adjacent to the aortic outline. The majority of thymomas are benign but 10–40% are malignant; 30–40% of patients with thymoma will suffer from myaesthenia gravis and 10% of patients with myaesthenia gravis will have a thymoma. Thymomas are also associated with red cell aplasia and hypogammaglobulinaemia. They are rare before the third decade.

## CASE 1.8 Cardiac failure

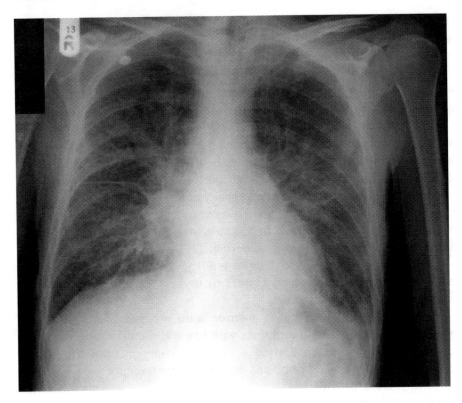

There is moderate cardiomegaly, the CTR being measured at '18 on 30' (measured from the actual radiograph). For further details see *Figure 1D*, p. 7. There is perihilar interstitial shadowing giving a typical 'bat's wing' appearance. In addition, there is upper lobe venous distension, and Kerley B lines are seen at both lung bases. These are the appearances of moderate congestive cardiac failure.

## Background

Cardiac enlargement is common in cardiac failure and indicates that the cardiac muscle is beginning to stretch. In association with cardiac enlargement, cardiac failure may then be classified radiologically as mild, moderate, or ultimately severe, by the presence of the following features as seen on an erect chest radiograph. These features correlate approximately with the right-sided pressure as indicated for each case.

*Mild cardiac failure:* there is upper lobe venous distension, whereby the upper lobe veins are larger than their lower lobe counterparts. This occurs because of relative hypoxaemia at the lung bases due to developing interstitial oedema, which thus results in blood flow diversion to the lung apices. The upper lobe veins distend as a result. Right atrial pressure is 10–15 mmHg.

*Moderate cardiac failure:* the development of further interstitial oedema results in poor definition of the vascular markings throughout the lung fields. These appearances are particularly marked adjacent to both hila, resulting in the classical 'bat's wing' appearance. At the lung bases this results in the development of Kerley B lines which occur due to the accumulation of fluid within the interlobular septa (*Figure 1.8a*). Pleural effusions may also be present, usually on the right side. Right atrial pressure is 15–20 mmHg.

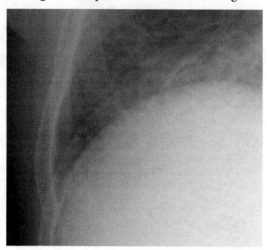

Figure 1.8a. Magnified view from CXR showing fluid within the interlobular septa, known as Kerley B lines.

*Severe cardiac failure:* this is seen as pulmonary oedema begins to develop. It is seen as bilateral patchy areas of air-space opacification due to fluid within the air spaces, and it is thus also referred to as alveolar opacification. Alveolar opacification is classically bilateral and symmetrical (cf. consolidation) and is also seen with the other features of cardiac failure as described above. Right atrial pressure is greater than 20 mmHg.

There may also be evidence of previous iatrogenic cardiac intervention, manifested by the presence of median sternotomy wires and coronary artery bypass graft (CABG) clips due to previous cardiac surgery, valve prosthesis or the presence of cardiac implants, defibrillators, or pacing devices (see *Case 1.19*).

## CASE 1.9 Pneumothorax

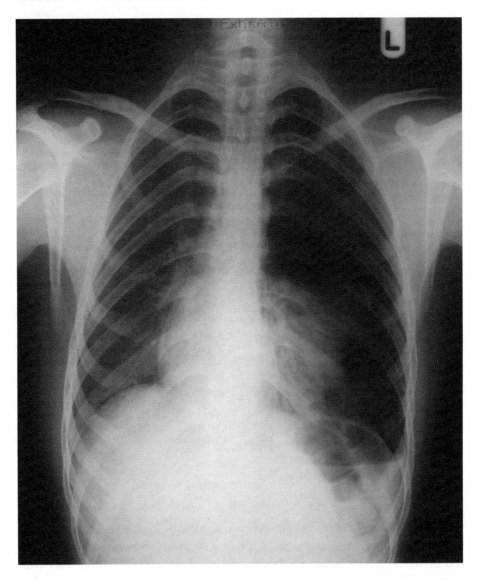

There is a complete collapse of the left lung and particular note is made that the mediastinum is shifted to the right side. These are the appearances of tension pneumothorax.

## Background

Pneumothorax is the presence of air between the layers of pleura (visceral and parietal) which are usually closely opposed, with only a trace of fluid normally present between them. It is easily seen in *Case 1.9*, but pneumothoraces can be very subtle, particularly if they are small and apical in position. Careful scrutiny for the lung edge may be necessary (*Figure 1.9a*), and thus the importance of 'the review areas' must be remembered (see p. 11).

Pneumothorax can occur spontaneously but also occurs in the following conditions:

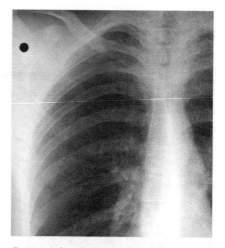

*Figure 1.9a. CXR showing a small right apical pneumothorax. Note the presence of the black dot on the right side of the film (actually red on the original radiograph). This was placed there by an experienced radiographer.*

- asthma
- COPD
- iatrogenic (eg. post-chest drain insertion, lung biopsy)
- trauma.

Treatment may be purely supportive, but air aspiration or ultimately chest drain insertion may be necessary. Referral is suggested to current British Thoracic Society guidelines. A small proportion of pneumothoraces may progress rapidly in size due to the so-called 'ball valve' phenomenon, whereby on each inhalation further air is sucked into the pleural space. This results in elevated pressure within the pleural space and is referred to as a tension pneumothorax.

The elevated pressure within the pleural space results in mediastinal shift to the opposite side, with compression of the opposite lung. In addition, the hemidiaphragm becomes everted. As mediastinal shift continues, there is increasing distortion of the great vessels, with compromise of blood returning to the heart. Compromise of cardiac return in association with developing hypoxaemia may lead to cardiac arrest.

A *tension pneumothorax* is a medical emergency and requires urgent intervention – if the patient is severely unwell, a standard intravenous cannula may be placed on the side of the pneumothorax in the second intercostal space and mid-clavicular line to allow immediate decompression prior to the introduction of a chest drain.

## CASE 1.10 Primary lung carcinoma

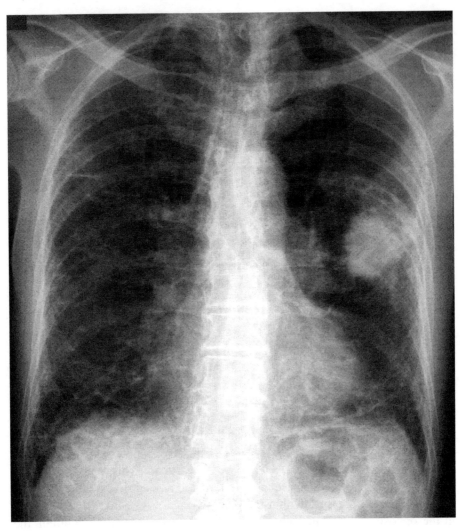

There is a poorly defined soft tissue mass at the left mid zone. This has an irregular spiculated edge and its appearances are those of a primary lung carcinoma. Note also the widespread linear change throughout both lungs, in keeping with idiopathic pulmonary fibrosis. These patients are at increased risk of developing primary bronchogenic carcinoma as is seen here.

## Background

This diagnosis is made by the presence of a soft tissue mass. The spiculated edge is typical of primary lung carcinoma. Sometimes the diagnosis is further confirmed by local invasion manifested by adjacent rib destruction. Further intrapulmonary deposits should be sought for, as should the presence of mediastinal lymphadenopathy. Occasionally, primary lung tumours may cavitate, particularly if they are of the squamous type (*Figure 1.10a*). These cases may be difficult to differentiate from necrotic lung abscess, but clinical correlation (eg. sepsis, raised white blood cell count) usually clarifies this.

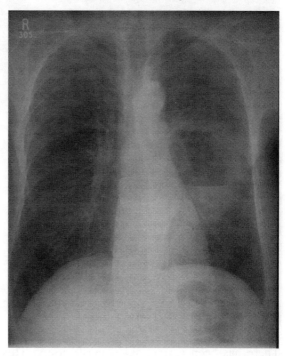

*Figure 1.10a. CXR showing large cavitating left mid-zone mass. This was histologically confirmed to be due to a squamous cell carcinoma.*

Staging is usually performed by CT whereby the whole chest and upper abdomen, including the adrenal glands and liver, is scanned. The tissue type is either obtained by biopsy via bronchoscopy (for centrally positioned lesions) or by CT-guided biopsy (for lesions closer to the lung periphery or at an intermediate position from which bronchoscopic washings have not been diagnostic). A CT scan demonstrating a primary lung malignancy is seen in *Case 5.15*, and an example of a CT-guided lung biopsy is shown in *Case 7.4*.

## CASE 1.11 Carcinoma of the breast and lung metastases

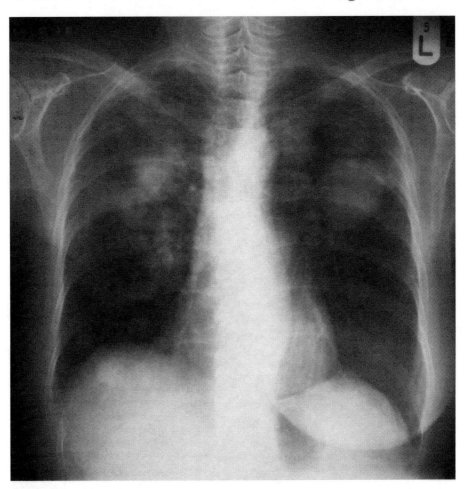

There has been a right-sided mastectomy. This is invariably performed for malignant breast disease. In addition, this film reveals the presence of multiple well-defined soft tissue masses throughout both lungs. These are in keeping with pulmonary metastases — presumably in this case from previous breast carcinoma. The bones appear normal with no evidence of bone deposits on this radiograph.

## Background

Checking for the presence and symmetry of breast tissue should be performed as a part of the review areas of the CXR (see p. 11), and abnormality is highly likely to indicate a history of breast malignancy.

Metastases to the lung parenchyma are typically seen as multiple well-defined soft tissue masses (cf. the spiculated edge of the solitary lung primary in *Case 1.10* on p. 34).

In cases such as *Case 1.11*, with a clear history of malignancy and secondary deposits, particular care should be taken to review the bones for further bone metastases.

Bone metastases from breast primary are typically sclerotic (see *Case 3.2*). In addition, there may have been previous radiotherapy. It is usually performed to the axillae, and there may therefore be evidence of radiation-induced lung fibrosis in this region. This is seen as a localised well-defined area of linear change that corresponds to the radiotherapy field.

Radiation osteonecrosis can also occur within the radiation field. This usually affects the angles of the ribs or the clavicle. Radiation osteonecrosis results in sclerotic bone changes very similar to the sclerotic changes due to bone metastases, and thus the history and the solitary nature of such a bone abnormality may be very important to help make this distinction.

## CASE 1.12 Dilated oesophagus

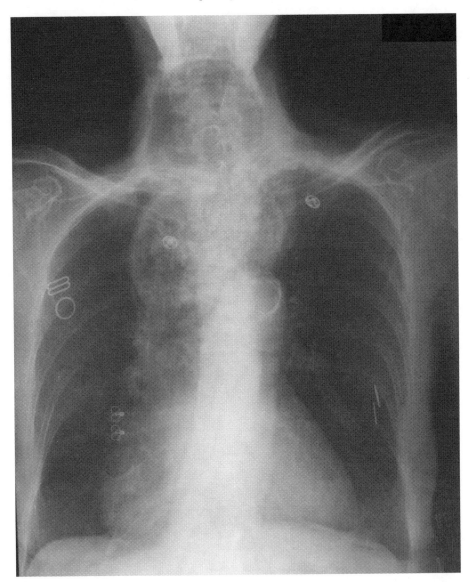

There is an air- and fluid-filled structure running vertically from the stomach as far as the superior mediastinum. This represents a dilated oesophagus. There is a differential diagnosis for these appearances as discussed below.

## Background

This is a difficult case, and at the time of the radiograph the final diagnosis was unclear. However, the patient was in her 80s. Further evaluation might be either by computed tomography, barium swallow, or endoscopy. Although barium swallow examinations are now dwindling in use (in comparison to endoscopy which enables biopsy of an obstructing lesion to be taken) swallow examinations are quick, effective and non-invasive. One was performed in the case above, and confirmed a dysmotile oesophagus with no evidence of obstructing lesion. A diagnosis of presbyoesophagus was made. Presbyoesophagus is an entity that results in dysmotility with no underlying systemic disorder, and typically occurs in the elderly.

A dilated oesophagus may be due to any of the following:

- *Obstructing lesion* to the lower oesophagus (eg. primary malignancy, benign tumour).
- *Achalasia* (neuromuscular contraction at the oesophagogastric junction).
- *Extrinsic compression* (eg. mediastinal lymph nodes).
- *Presbyoesophagus* (as above).
- *Dysmotile oesophagus* secondary to connective tissue diseases (eg. scleroderma).
- *Primary dysmotility* not related to age or underlying connective tissue disease.
- *Foreign body* (eg. food bolus).

## CASE 1.13 Pleural effusion

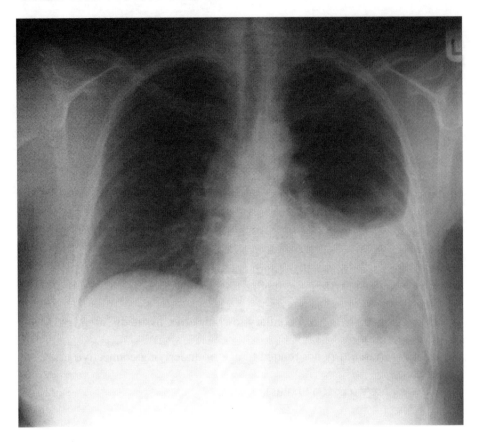

There is complete loss of the left costophrenic angle, with uniform density also extending up the lateral chest wall, and a meniscus sign is seen on the left lateral chest wall. The appearances are those of a large left-sided pleural effusion. There is no evidence of associated mediastinal shift thus suggesting that there must also be a degree of associated pulmonary collapse. In this case, note the absence of the left breast and surgical clips in the left axilla which suggest a history of previous breast malignancy and axillary lymph node clearance. This is therefore probably a malignant effusion, which could be confirmed by aspiration and cytological analysis.

## Background

Pleural effusion collects in the most dependent parts of the chest, and thus on the erect CXR will be seen to obscure the costophrenic angle, forming a meniscus up the lateral chest wall. The fluid is seen as uniform fluid density unless there is associated collapse or consolidation of the adjacent lung. If the pleural effusion is of moderate or large size, it usually causes mass effect and may result in collapse of adjacent lung or mediastinal shift. Conversely, if there is a large pleural effusion and no evidence of mediastinal shift, then this strongly suggests a degree of lung collapse (although this collapse may of course be due to mass effect secondary to the fluid rather than the primary cause).

Pleural fluid may be divided into transudate or exudate depending on its protein content:

* transudate: less than 30 mg protein/litre
* exudate: more than 30 mg protein/litre.

There is no difference radiographically between transudate and exudate, although, of course, the underlying cause may be seen (eg. cardiac failure, pneumonia, or malignancy).

Causes of transudate include:

* cardiac failure
* renal failure
* hepatic failure
* hypoproteinaemic states.

Causes of exudate include:

* infection (bacterial, viral or TB)
* malignancy
* pulmonary infarction
* pancreatitis.

## CASE 1.14 Extraluminal gas

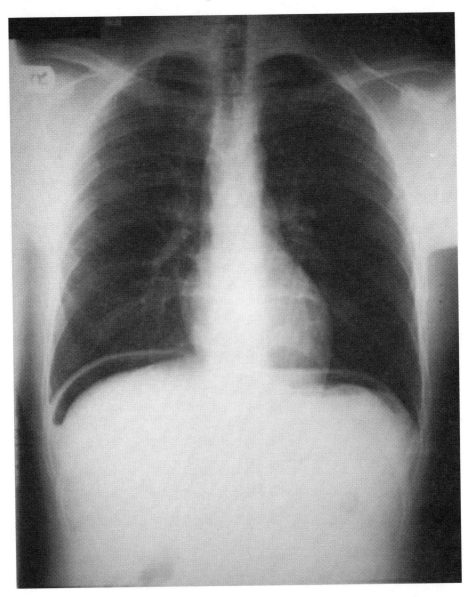

Erect chest radiograph showing lucent arcs under both hemidiaphragms in keeping with free intraperitoneal gas.

## Background

This occurs due to leakage of gas through a perforation of a gas-containing viscus (ie. bowel) into the peritoneal space. Gas is best demonstrated as a lucent arc under the hemidiaphragms on an erect chest radiograph or erect abdominal film. True free gas must not be confused with intraluminal bowel gas within a bowel loop that has come to lie between the liver and the right hemidiaphragm – so-called colonic interposition or Chilidaiti syndrome (*Figure 1.14a*). This can be differentiated from true free gas by the presence of haustra. The importance of the erect CXR in a patient with an acute abdomen cannot be over-stressed. The CXR should be performed after the patient has sat erect for 10–15 minutes to ensure that any free gas present rises to the subdiaphragmatic area. This technique can show as little as 1 mL of free gas.

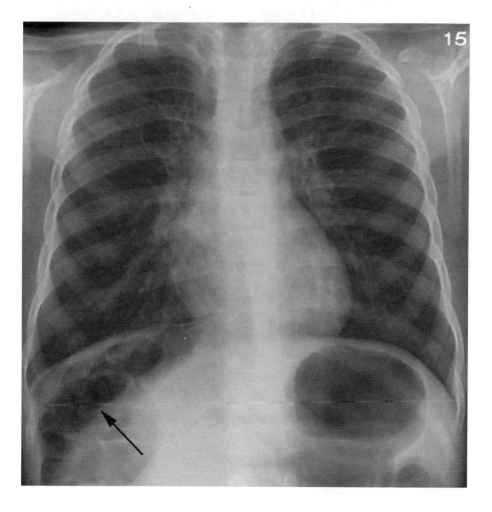

*Figure 1.14a. CXR demonstrating Chilidaiti syndrome. Note the presence of haustra (arrow).*

If the erect CXR fails to clearly show free gas, or if the patient is unable to sit upright, a right-side-up lateral decubitus film (where the patient lies on their left side for the exposure) is performed. This will show any free gas within the peritoneal space, and by lying right side uppermost it will not be confused with air within the stomach (see *Figure 1.14b*).

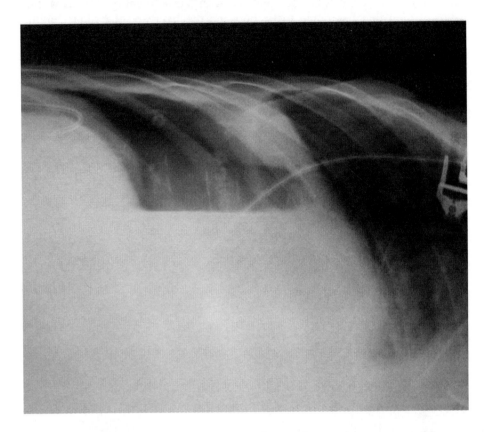

Figure 1.14b. Right-side-up lateral decubitus film confirming the presence of free gas in a patient too unwell to sit up for an erect CXR.

Finally, free gas should not be confused with gas within the stomach. It will usually be obvious due to the thickness of the overlying soft tissue 'arc' which constitutes both diaphragm and stomach wall, and by the presence of a fluid level within the stomach itself (*Figure 1.14c*).

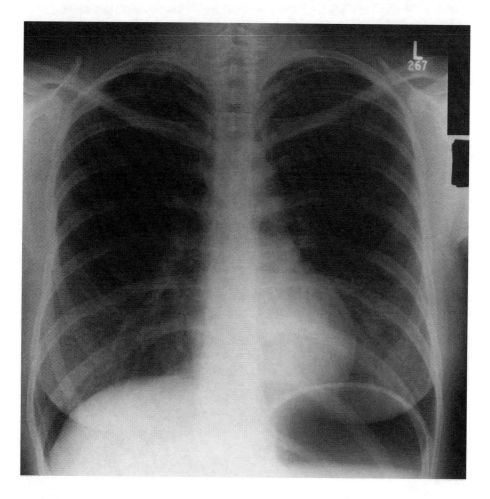

Figure 1.14c. CXR showing prominent gas bubble within the stomach.

## CASE 1.15 Pneumonia

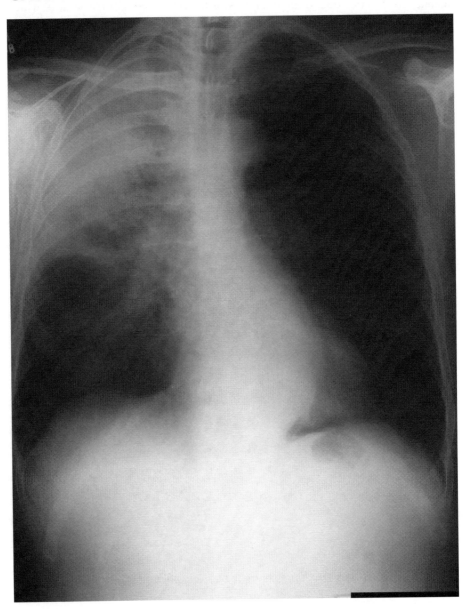

There is volume loss within the right upper lobe due to a combination of collapse and consolidation. An air bronchogram is seen within the area of consolidation. The appearances are in keeping with collapse and consolidation due to pneumonia.

## Background

Air-space changes are classically poorly defined (easily remembered as 'cloud like') and if persistent aeration is present within the bronchi, then these air-filled tubular structures may be seen as they pass through the area of consolidation. This is called an 'air bronchogram'.

Air-space changes occur due to the air within normally aerated lung being replaced by fluid or cellular infiltrate. Fluid may take the form of *pus* (in cases of pneumonia, as in *Figure 1.15a*), *transudate* or *exudate* (in cases of cardiac, renal or hepatic failure), *blood* (due to trauma), or more rarely *cellular infiltrate* (alveolar cell carcinoma). It is apparent that there is a wide differential diagnosis of air-space opacification. The case shown here was known to be coughing up large amounts of phlegm, and was pyrexial with an elevated white blood cell count. The appearances are thus entirely in keeping with the suspected clinical diagnosis of pneumonia.

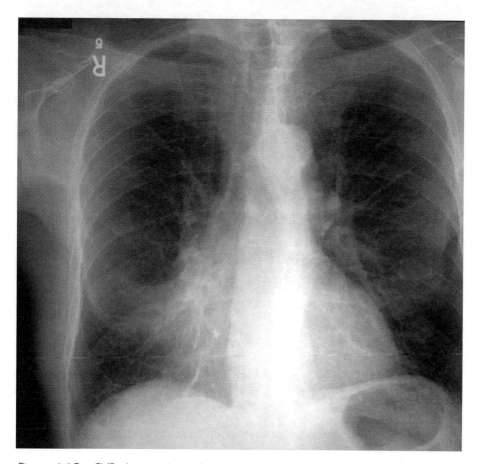

*Fig.ure 1.15a. CXR showing loss of the normal right heart border and opacification in this area due to consolidation because of pneumonia in the right middle lobe.*

Pneumonia may be localised to any anatomical lobe, and if there is associated volume loss this suggests there is a degree of lobar collapse; hence the ubiquitous, but not always accurate, term of 'collapse/consolidation'. An example of this is given by the classial 'sail' sign as shown in *Figure 1.15b*. An example of upper lobar consolidation is shown in *Figure 1.15c*. Aspiration pneumonia tends to occur to the right lower lobe, since the right main bronchus is orientated more vertically than its left-sided counterpart (*Figure 1.15d*).

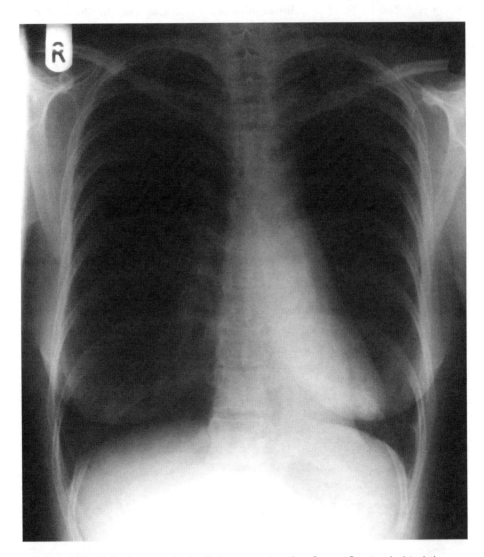

*Figure 1.15b. CXR showing the 'sail' sign – a triangle of opacification behind the cardiac silhouette. This is due to left lower lobe collapse.*

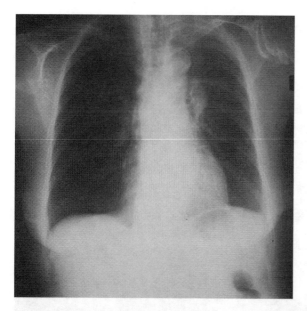

*Figure 1.15c. CXR showing a veil-like opacification of the left upper and middle zones. There is persistent aeration adjacent to the aortic knuckle (the so-called 'luft [air] sickle' sign). This is the appearance of left upper lobe consolidation.*

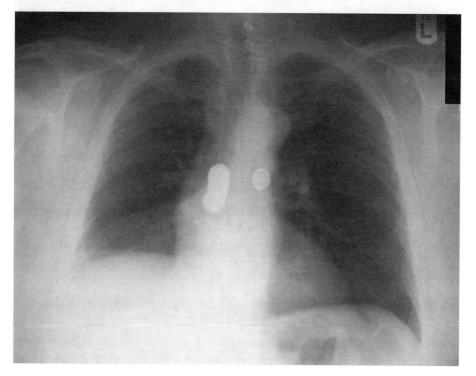

*Figure 1.15d. CXR of a male patient who has been performing a party trick of catching not peanuts in his mouth but five-pence coins. He repeated this eleven times, and aspirated nine of them (45p) into his right main bronchus, and only two of them into the left side! Remember aspiration is more likely to occur to the right main bronchus. Previously published in British Medical Journal, 2002, 325: 1310.*

## CASE 1.16 Chronic obstructive pulmonary disease

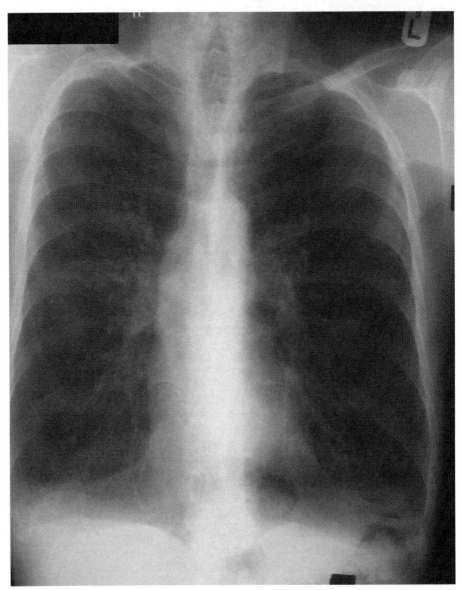

There is evidence of hyperinflation, with flattening of both hemidiaphragms, and apparent narrowing and elongation of the mediastinum. There is coarsening of the lung markings, and several bullae are also seen. There is tethering and fibrosis at the lung bases and apices in keeping with previous infections. The pulmonary arteries are centrally enlarged, in keeping with pulmonary arterial hypertension due to chronic hypoxaemia. These are the appearances of chronic obstructive pulmonary disease (COPD) or emphysema.

## Background

The changes described above are typical of COPD. These patients are susceptible to recurrent chest infections, and particular evaluation should be made for areas of active consolidation, or for pneumothorax which may give rise to an acute deterioration requiring treatment. Further to this, these patients are usually long-term smokers, and as such are at increased risk of lung cancer.

The analysis of the acute film is often helped by comparing it with previous radiographs to evaluate if subtle changes were actually present previously, and thus whether there has been any suspicious interval development. Alternatively, it may be noted that a potential area of consolidation was present many years previously, and has not changed in the interim; thus being of doubtful significance.

Finally, a dense area of opacification may be difficult to differentiate between air-space change (and thus pneumonia) or soft tissue mass (and thus malignancy). Obviously, this is an important differentiation to make, and thus either antibiotic treatment and a subsequent CXR may be performed, or if there is serious concern as to whether malignancy is present, then the patient may be referred directly for a CT scan of the chest.

Assessment for hemidiaphragmatic flattening is shown in *Figure 1.16a*.

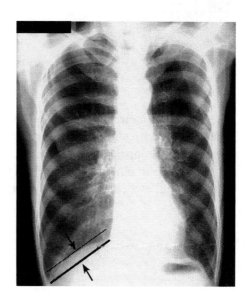

*Figure 1.16a. CXR showing how to assess diapragmatic flattening. A line is drawn from the cardiophrenic angle to the costophrenic angle. Flattening is said to occur if the arc of the diaphragm is less than 1.5 cm from this line.*

## CASE 1.17 Pulmonary embolus

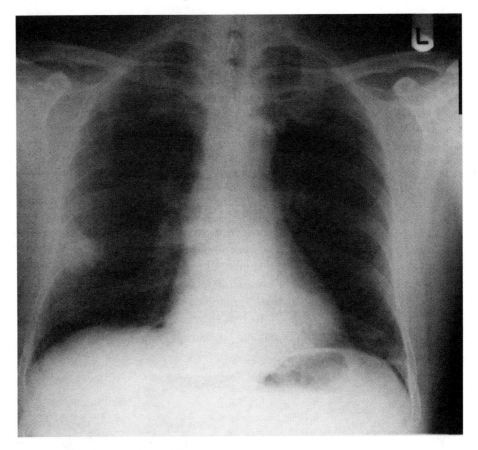

There is linear atelectasis at the left lung base. In addition, there is peripheral triangular opacification at the right mid zone which is suggestive of pulmonary infarct. These appearances are not specific and may be due to infection or infarction due to pulmonary embolus (PE). Indeed, the linear collapse may be longstanding, and clinical correlation is particularly important in this case.

## Background

Pulmonary emboli can give rise to a variety of appearances on the plain chest radiograph (the first three listed here are most usually seen):

* normal appearances
* pleural effusion
* linear atelectasis
* oligaemic segment
* wedge-shaped peripheral pulmonary infarction
* pulmonary plethora in the segments of lung which maintain their perfusion
* enlargement of the central pulmonary vessels due to acute pulmonary hypertension.

The most likely appearance, however, of PE is of the normal chest radiograph, or presence of pleural effusion and atelectasis. Clinical correlation with evaluation of radiograph findings is always important, but this is particularly so in cases of suspected pulmonary emboli because the changes on the CXR are non-specific, and the potential risk of non-treatment is high.

## The evaluation of suspected PE

Until recently, radionuclide imaging has often been the usual examination performed in the evaluation of suspected PE. This is the VQ scan (where V is for ventilation and Q is for perfusion) see *Figure 1.17a*. Isotopes of technetium and krypton are injected intravenously and inhaled, respectively. The lungs are then imaged using a gamma camera. Acute PE will give a mismatch of the perfusion and ventilation patterns, that is the lung segment containing emboli will have decreased blood flow to it, but will still be ventilated. However, this examination only gives the probability of emboli as low or high, and many scans are indeterminate. A low or high probability scan is only correct in 90% of cases, and thus up to 10% are incorrect. More invasive techniques, including pulmonary artery angiography, have therefore been used in some centres. They involve placing a catheter in the right side of the heart via the femoral vein. Radiographic contrast is then injected into the pulmonary circulation and a PE is seen as a filling defect within the pulmonary circulation with an associated oligaemic peripheral segment.

CT pulmonary angiography (CTPA) is now generally accepted as the examination of choice in cases of suspected PE. This involves contrast injection to the antecubital fossa through a standard intravenous cannula. A CT scan of the lungs is then performed which is timed to coincide with maximal contrast flow through the pulmonary arteries. Pulmonary emboli are seen as filling defects within the pulmonary vessels (see *Figure 1.17b*). CTPA is fast, non-invasive, and is not only more accurate in detecting PEs (95–99%), but will also detect other pulmonary pathology.

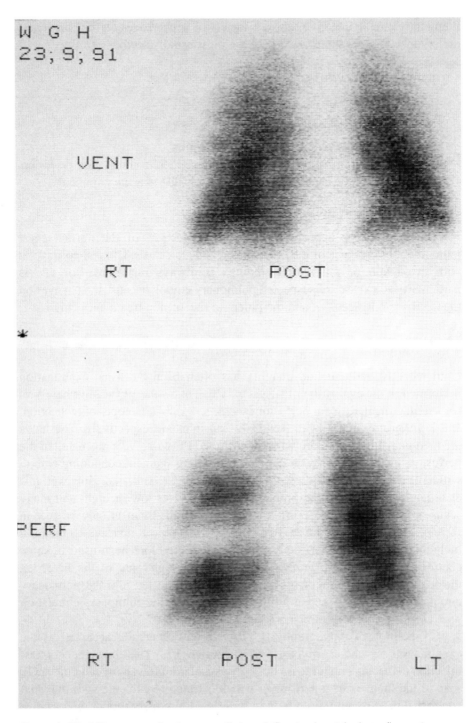

*Figure 1.17a. VQ scan confirming a perfusion defect in the right lung (lower image, PERF), with normal ventilation (upper image, VENT). The appearances are in keeping with pulmonary embolus.*

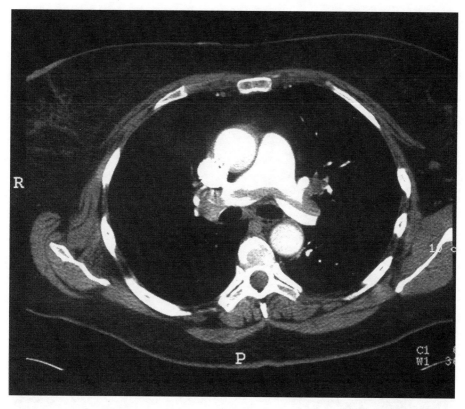

*Figure 1.17b. CT pulmonary angiogram (CTPA) showing filling defects bridging both main pulmonary arteries in keeping with saddle pulmonary embolus.*

## CASE 1.18 Mitral valve disease

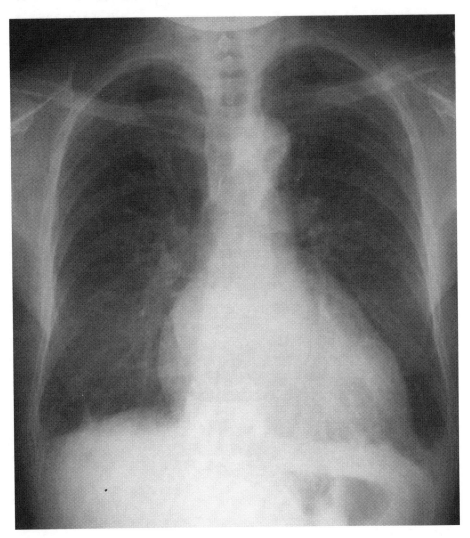

The heart is enlarged, and there is evidence of left atrial enlargement (seen as a bulge to the left heart border, and a double shadow seen behind the right side of the heart). There is associated congestive cardiac failure. These are the appearances of cardiac failure, with associated mitral valve disease causing left atrial enlargement.

## Background

Mitral valve disease is usually a combination of stenosis and regurgitation and results in dilation of the left atrium. As a result, the left atrium is seen as a double right-heart border, enlargement of the left atrial appendage, and possibly splaying of the carina (since the left atrium enlarges into the space below and between the left and right main bronchi). See the annotated CXR below (*Figure 1.18a*). Ultimately, mitral valve disease may lead to congestive cardiac failure. These appearances can be confirmed by echocardiography. Pulmonary venous hypertension due to mitral valve disease may also result in haemoptysis which, if chronic, may occasionally calcify, to be seen as multiple calcified pulmonary nodules (see *Case 1.3*).

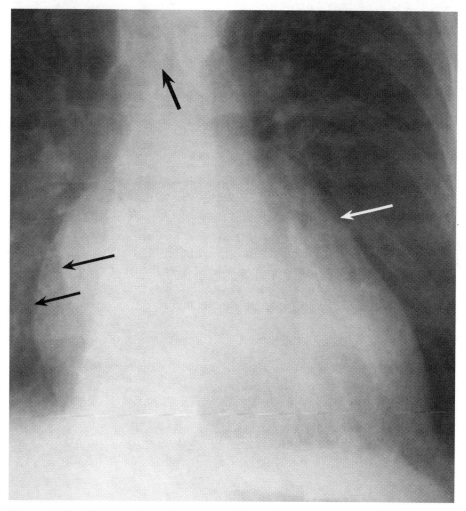

*Figure 1.18a. CXR showing enlargement of the left atrium causing double right heart border (thin black arrows), enlarged left atrial appendage (white arrow), and splaying of the carina (thick black arrow).*

## CASE 1.19 Implants and evidence of previous interventions

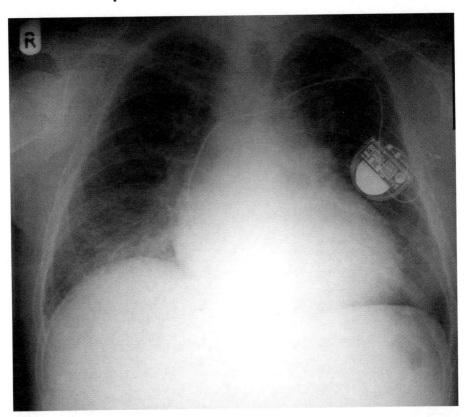

This is a chest radiograph of a patient who has median sternotomy wires and arterial clips in keeping with CABG. In addition there is a single-chamber pacemaker *in situ*, with its wire tip projected over the right ventricular apex. Furthermore, there is also evidence of cardiomegaly and upper lobe venous distension, in keeping with moderate cardiac failure.

## Background

There is a potential for numerous iatrogenic wires, lines, tubes (*Figure 1.19a*), valves, clips, and other implantation devices (defibrillators or pacemakers). These may be confusing unless you've seen them before.

The appearances in *Case 1.19* are those of the commonly performed median sternotomy, which has been carried out in order to perform CABG (often pronounced *cabbage*). The wires are used to close the medial incision through the sternum. In addition, a single-chamber pacemaker has been implanted with its wire tip correctly positioned within the muscle of the right ventricular apex. Dual-chamber pacemakers are also commonly seen, with two wires; one seen to lie as above, and the other curved and lying to abut the muscle of the right atrium.

Examples of aortic and mitral valve replacements are shown in *Figures 1.19b* and *1.19c*. Note that the right-sided heart valves, the tricuspid and pulmonary valves, are not commonly replaced.

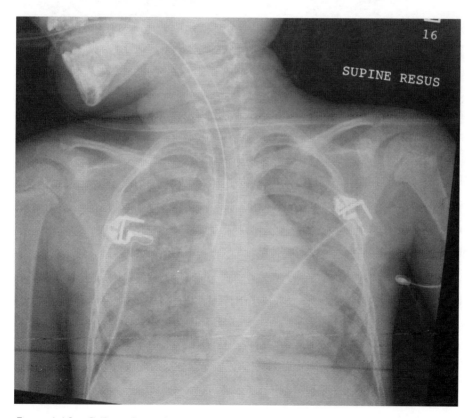

*Figure 1.19a. CXR performed supine in the resuscitation room of the accident and emergency department. There are ECG leads applied to the chest, and an endotracheal tube (ETT) is seen within the trachea (the tip is actually positioned within the right main bronchus and it should be withdrawn 3–4 cm).*

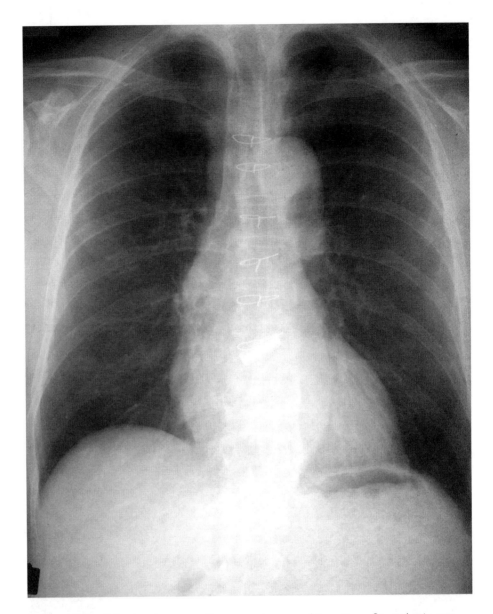

Figure 1.19b. CXR showing a median sternotomy and insertion of prosthetic aortic valve (note its position at the aortic root, and that it lies within the horizontal plane).

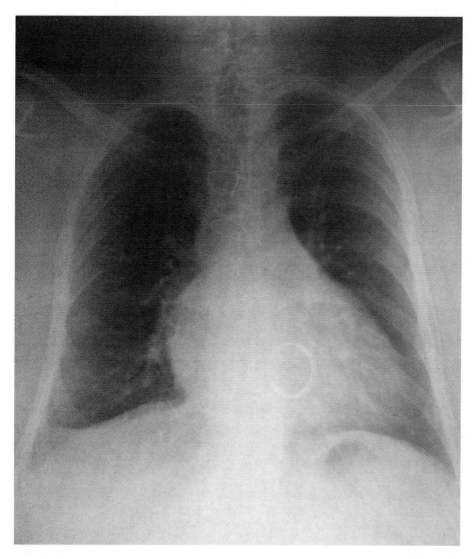

*Fig.ure 1.19c. CXR showing a median sternotomy and insertion of prosthetic mitral valve (note its position more centrally within the cardiac outline, and its vertical plane allowing one 'to see through the valve' from the left ventricle into the left atrium).*

## CASE 1.20 Bronchiectasis

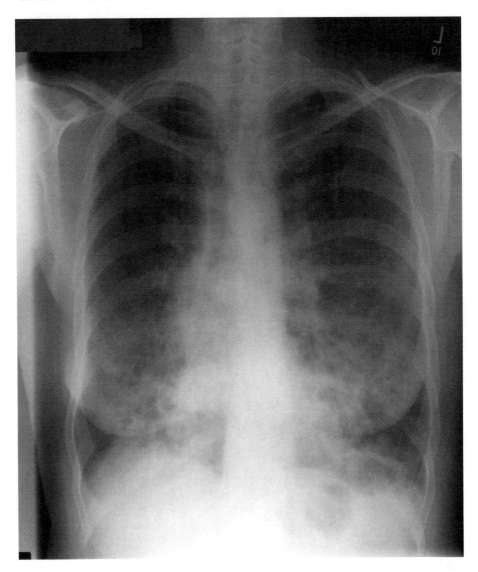

There are multiple areas of peribronchial thickening, and cystic changes predominantly at both lung bases. These changes are in keeping with bronchiectasis.

## Background

Bronchiectasis means dilation of the airways, which becomes clinically significant as it may predispose to recurrent infections, haemopytsis, and ultimately pulmonary hypertension. The causes include:

* post-infective (eg. TB, whooping cough, measles)
* cystic fibrosis
* obstruction (eg. an inhaled peanut or a lymph node)
* congenital (eg. Kartagener syndrome).

On the CXR, bronchiectasis results in thickening and dilation of the bronchial walls, resulting in tramline shadows. The bronchi are dilated when their diameter exceeds that of the adjacent pulmonary artery. The bronchi may also become fluid filled. Ultimately cysts may form within the lung, and these may fill with fluid if they become infected. If these appearances are seen in a young patient, the likely cause is cystic fibrosis. Always check for the presence of dextrocardia since this is likely to indicate the patient is suffering from Kartagener syndrome (the immotile cilia syndrome manifested by bronchiectasis, dextrocardia, and recurrent sinusitis). In chronic cases, pulmonary hypertension may develop with enlargement of the central pulmonary arteries, and basal lung fibrosis.

After the initial CXR, the radiographic examination of choice in the evaluation of bronchiectasis is high-resolution computed tomography (HRCT) of the chest (see *Figures 1.20a* and *1.20b*). This involves narrow-section CT slices (usually a thickness of 1–2 mm rather than the standard for CT chest of 3–10 mm). In addition, since bronchiectasis is usually a diffuse disease, these narrow slices can be performed non-contiguously (eg. a 1.5 mm slice every 15 mm of lung) as this will decrease the radiation exposure to the patient. Remember, therefore, that the entire volume of the lungs is not being scanned with HRCT, and thus mass lesions may not be visualised if they happen to lie between the slices taken. Accordingly, if there is a possibility of mass, lymphadenopathy or other focal lung pathology, then a standard CT protocol of the chest may be needed in addition to HRCT.

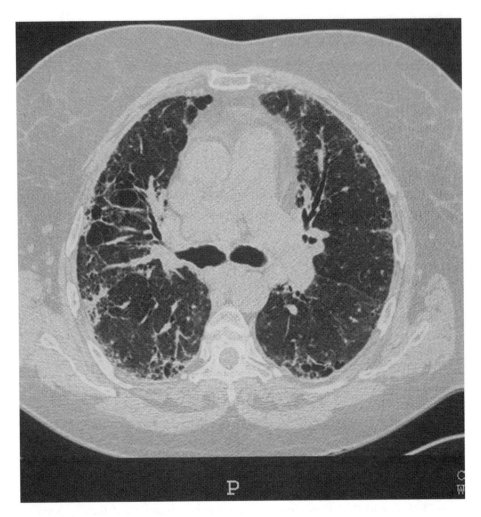

*Figure 1.20a. High-resolution CT (HRCT) showing peribronchial thickening and dilation with bronchi seen in the plane of the scan.*

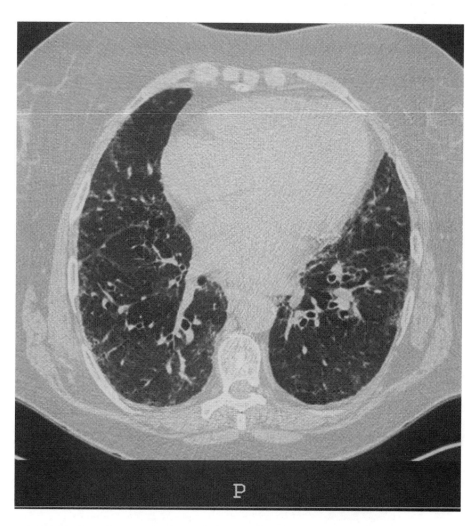

*Figure 1.20b. High-resolution CT (HRCT) showing peribronchial thickening and dilation with the scan passing through the bronchi which appear as rings.*

## CASE 1.21 Coarctation

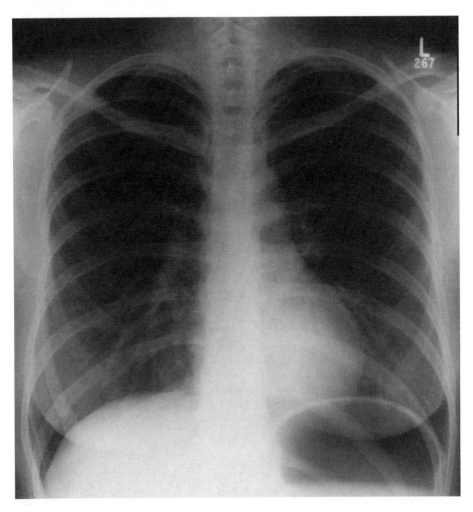

There may be evidence of subtle inferior rib notching bilaterally, and the aortic arch is of narrow calibre. The appearances are in keeping with coarctation of the aorta, and further evaluation with CT or MRI of the aorta is indicated.

## Background

Coarctation of the aorta involves narrowing of the aortic lumen, usually just below the origin of the left subclavian artery. This results in the classical radiofemoral delay in pulses, with hypertension in both arms. Collateral blood flow therefore develops through the intercostal arteries. These vessels lie within the subcostal grooves beneath each rib, and their distension results in notching to the inferior rib surface (remember, whenever passing a needle into the chest to always do so just above a rib in order to avoid these structures). The ascending aorta is often dilated, and the aorta distal to the coarct is narrow. The actual site of the coarct may also be seen as a notch to the aortic lumen. There may be associated left ventricular distension and possibly signs of cardiac failure.

Remember that as well as the intercostal artery, the intercostal vein and nerve run within the subcostal groove, and therefore pathology of *each* of these structures may cause inferior rib notching (*Figure 1.21a*) thus:

* intercostal artery – coarctation of the aorta or aortic thrombosis
* intercostal vein – superior vena cava (SVC) or subclavian vein obstruction
* intercostal nerve – neurofibromatosis.

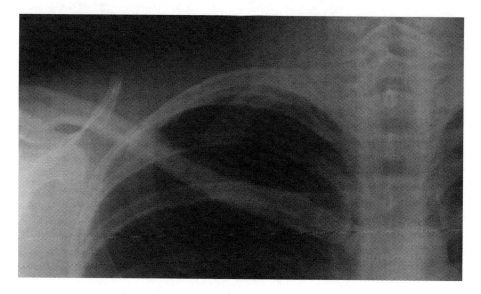

Figure 1.21a. Magnified view from CXR showing inferior rib notching.

# Section 2

# The Abdominal Radiograph

# Introduction

The abdominal radiograph is commonly requested by surgical and A & E staff. However, its interpretation is often basic and is purely to determine whether the patient is suffering from intestinal obstruction. As with other radiograph interpretation, the abdominal radiograph requires a methodical assessment of all aspects of the film. A system of analysis should include not only the bowel gas pattern, but also review of the soft tissue outlines and bone.

### Bowel gas pattern

The initial AXR assessment invariably involves evaluation of the bowel gas pattern. Before it is possible to determine if a particular loop of bowel is dilated, one must first ascertain if it is small bowel or colon. The distribution, calibre and mucosal pattern of the bowel are all important in making this distinction (see *Table 2.1*).

## Table 2.1 Differentiation of small and large bowel

| Feature | Small bowel | Large bowel |
|---|---|---|
| Distribution | Central | Peripheral |
| Mucosal pattern | Valvulae conniventes crossing the width of the bowel | Haustra do not cross the entire width |
| Calibre | Jejunum 3.5 cm (max) Ileum 2.5 cm (max) | 5.5 cm (max) |
| Number of loops | Many | Few, rarely seen |
| Presence of solid faeces | Absent | Present |
| Radius of curvature | Small | Large |

There is rarely enough gas in the small bowel to see more than short segments of mucosal outline, but the transverse mucosal folds (valvulae conniventes) of the small bowel are closer together and cross the entire bowel lumen (*Figure 2A*). This can sometimes give rise to a 'stack of coins' appearance. The distal ileum can appear smooth when dilated, which may further complicate interpretation. Small bowel is generally centrally positioned, and the loops are more numerous and demonstrate a tighter radius of curvature than those in the large bowel. The presence of solid faeces is an indicator of large bowel, which can also be recognised by the incomplete haustral band crossing the colonic gas shadow (*Figure 2B*). Haustra are usually present in the ascending and transverse colon but may be absent from the splenic flexure and descending colon.

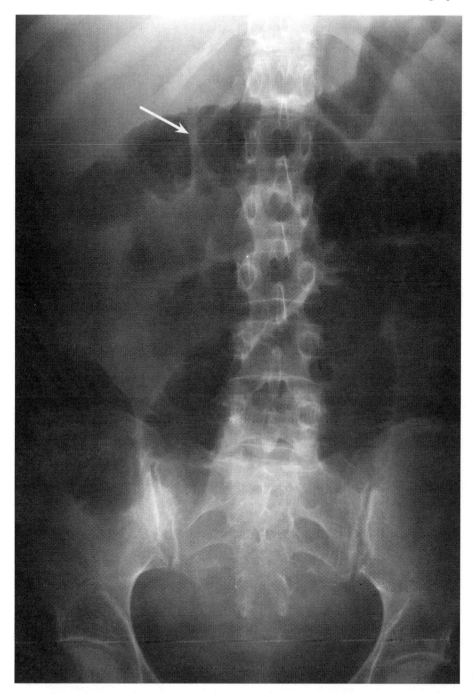

*Figure 2A. Plain abdominal radiograph showing the valvulae conniventes (arrow) crossing the entire bowel lumen.*

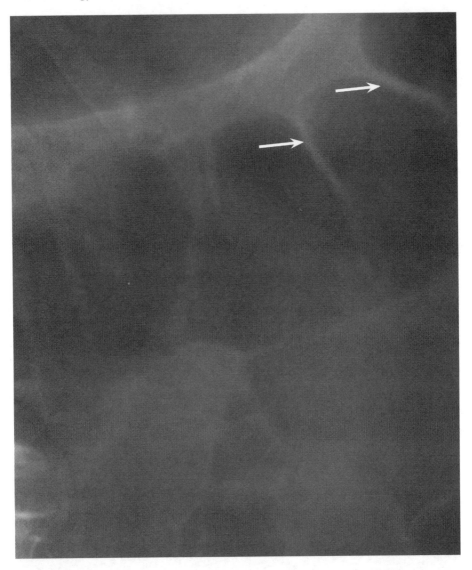

*Figure 2B. Magnified view from plain abdominal radiograph. The haustra are shown (arrows) and are seen not to cross the bowel lumen.*

When a loop has been assessed to be small bowel or colon, the direct measurement of the bowel diameter will give a reasonable assessment of the degree of dilatation. Small bowel maximum calibre is 3.5 cm in the jejunum and 2.5 cm in the ileum. Large bowel calibre can measure up to 5.5 cm in diameter. Diameters significantly greater than this may be at risk of perforation. Caecal perforation is a risk with diameters greater than 9 cm.

After the bowel gas pattern has been evaluated, the soft tissue outlines should be examined.

## Soft tissue outlines

The normal visceral anatomy of liver edge, renal outlines and splenic tip may be seen. These structures are particularly well outlined if the patient has a significant amount of intraperitoneal fat, which helps to demarcate soft tissue planes. The aortic wall is seen if it is calcified, and its normal diameter (even allowing for radiographic magnification) rarely exceeds 2.5 cm. Further vascular calcification may be seen, particularly within the splenic vessels, as serpiginous tramlines of calcific density in the left upper quadrant. Calcified renal tract stones or, more rarely, gallstones may also be seen.

An abnormal soft tissue mass or abscess may be seen in addition to these structures. If there is a suspicion of an abnormal soft tissue mass, an ultrasound, or CT scan may be indicated. An abscess classically has a rather heterogenous density due to gas, pus and necrotic tissue within it. In addition, the position of displaced bowel within the abdomen may be indirect evidence of abdominal or pelvic mass.

A specific evaluation should then be made for extraluminal gas, abnormal areas of calcification and the bones. Evidence of previous surgery may also give clues as to current pathology.

## Bones

The bones of the spine and pelvis should also be examined; a bone lesion may be evidence of metastatic disease from an already noted suspicious mass lesion and be highly relevant in a patient already known to have a malignant primary. Vertebral collapse due to metastatic or osteoporotic disease can be easily overlooked, and this may be the cause of radicular pain mimicking pain of abdominal origin. Collectively, these features combine for final interpretation and the formulation of a differential diagnosis.

---

### Key points of the abdominal radiograph

- Remember to analyse soft tissues outlines, bowel gas patterns, and other features on the film.
- Discriminate between small and large bowel.
- Know the normal bowel calibre.
- Examine bones of spine and pelvis.

## CASE 2.1 Small bowel obstruction

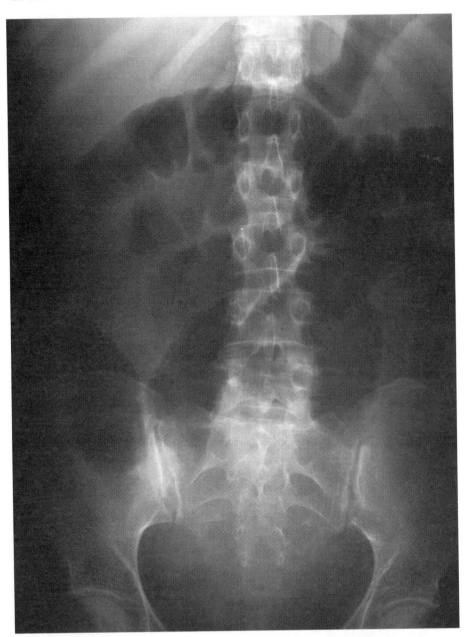

There are multiple loops of dilated, centrally positioned bowel. These contain valvulae conniventes, so they represent small bowel. The diameters of the loops of bowel in this case are in excess of 3 cm, meaning they are dilated. These are, therefore, the appearances of small bowel obstruction.

## Background

Mechanical small bowel obstruction (SBO) results in multiple loops of dilated, centrally positioned bowel, often with tight radius of curvature. A paucity of large bowel gas distal to the site of obstruction may also be a helpful sign.

The small bowel loops are clearly seen in this case because they are gas filled, but the appearances can be much more subtle if they are fluid filled. In these cases only a few gas bubbles may be seen, trapped against the mucosal surface, resulting in the so-called 'string of beads' sign. If there is real doubt, an erect film may clearly demonstrate multiple air-fluid levels, but this is usually waived in favour of CT if there is clinical doubt as to the diagnosis (*Figure 2.1a*). SBO usually occurs due to post-surgical adhesions (look for surgical clips) or inguinal hernia (look for gas overlying the inguinal canals) (see *Case 2.11*). Other causes include:

- Stricture such as Crohn's disease, secondary to radiotherapy, or rarely infections (eg. TB, *Yersinia*).
- Gallstone ileus.

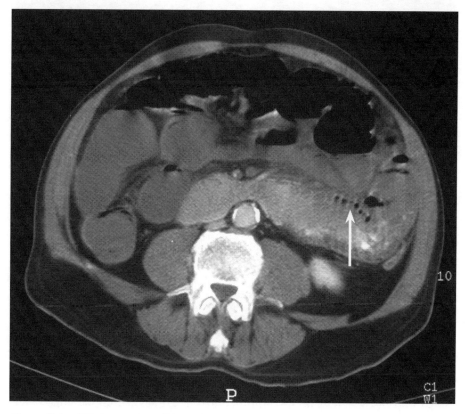

*Figure 2.1a. CT showing small bowel obstruction and 'string of beads' sign (arrow).*

## CASE 2.2 Gallstone ileus

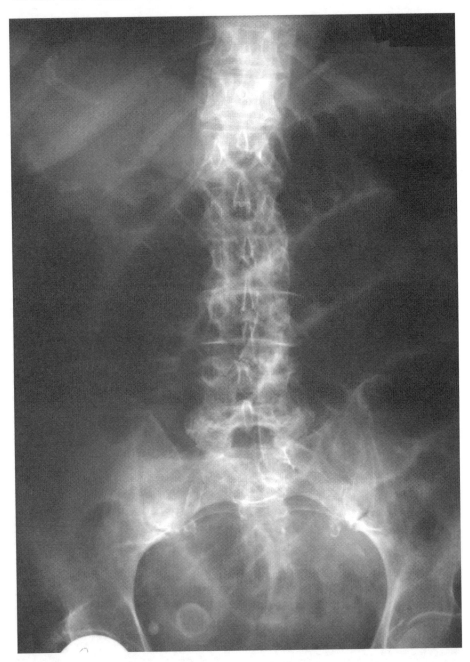

There are multiple loops of dilated, centrally positioned small bowel. There is a radio-opaque calculus in the right iliac fossa, and gas within the biliary tree. The appearances are in keeping with gallstone ileus.

## Background

Gallstone ileus is a rare cause of small bowel obstruction, which can give a classical appearance on AXR. It occurs when a large gallstone passes from the biliary tree into the small bowel, where it comes to rest at the ileocaecal valve causing small bowel obstruction. If the stone is calcified then it may be seen in the right iliac fossa. In addition, the stone's passage or erosion from the biliary tree into the duodenum may allow reflux of gas back into the biliary tree to give a branching low-density pattern in the right upper quadrant (*Figure 2.2a*).

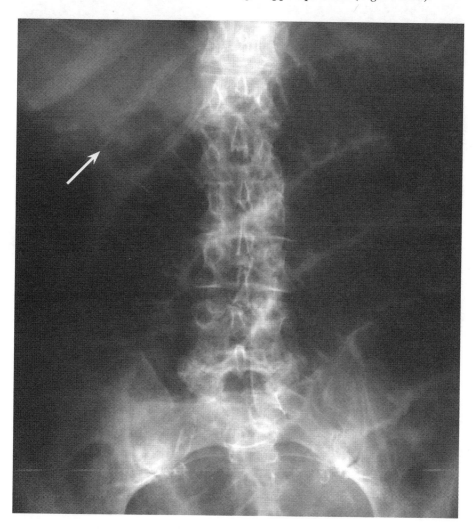

*Figure 2.2a. Magnified view of right upper quadrant showing the branching pattern of gas within the biliary tree (arrow).*

## CASE 2.3 Large bowel obstruction

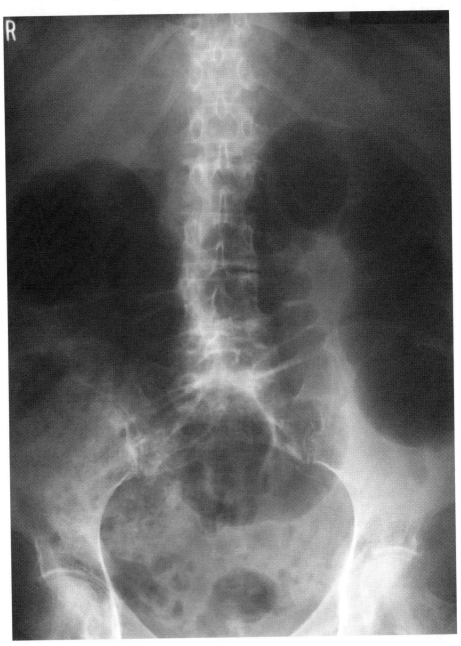

There is dilated large bowel seen as far as a soft tissue mass in the left inguinal fossa. These are the appearances of large bowel obstruction, probably due to colonic carcinoma. Remember to evaluate the film in such cases for evidence of metastatic disease (eg. bone deposits).

## Background

The dilatation of the large bowel is seen as far as the level of obstruction, where the bowel calibre is seen to be narrowed, or the causative lesion is seen (eg. bowel-related primary malignancy). There may be accompanying small-bowel dilation if the ileocaecal valve is incompetent. Indeed, ileocaecal valve incompetence can result in caecal decompression, thus reducing the probability of caecal perforation. The presence of such a mass might be confirmed by either enema examination or sigmoidoscopy. A CT scan of such a case would not only confirm the presence of a mass (*Figure 2.3a*), but would also effectively stage the tumour prior to treatment.

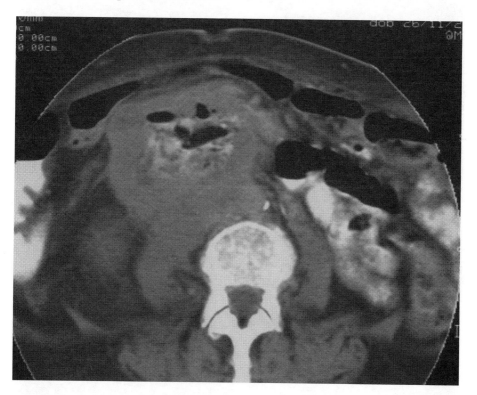

*Figure 2.3a. Computed tomographic scan demonstrating a mass in the transverse colon in keeping with colonic cancer.*

## CASE 2.4 Toxic megacolon

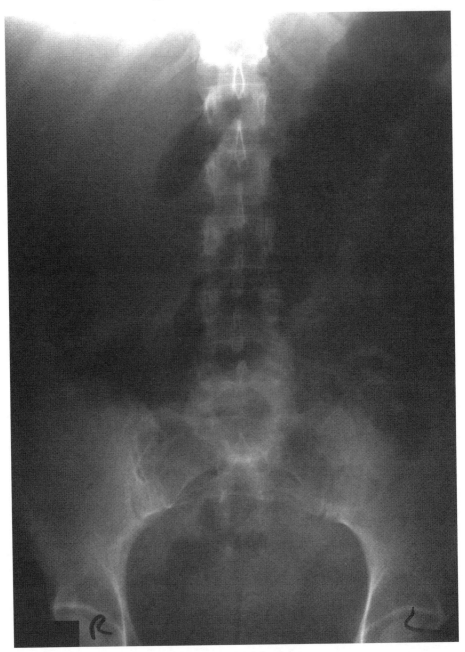

The transverse colon is gas filled and mildly dilated, with poor definition of the mucosal outline and 'thumb-printing' indicating mucosal oedema and ulceration. These are the appearances of toxic megacolon. Repeat abdominal radiographs are recommended to monitor the degree of dilatation. An erect chest radiograph is probably also indicated to exclude perforation.

### Background

Toxic megacolon may be the diagnosis when the diameter of the colon exceeds 5.5 cm. In order to differentiate these appearances from simple uncomplicated large bowel obstruction, the additional features of blurring of the mucosal outline and thumb-printing should be present. The later features indicate mucosal oedema and ulceration. Toxic megacolon most commonly occurs in inflammatory bowel disease (Crohn's disease or ulcerative colitis). This may have been revealed in the history.

Toxic megacolon may also occur in cases of ischaemic bowel. This often occurs due to thromboembolism and thus note should be made if the patient is in atrial fibrillation. Ischaemic colitis classically occurs at the junction of the middle and distal thirds of the transverse colon, since this is the watershed area between blood supplies from the superior and inferior mesenteric arteries, respectively.

## CASE 2.5 Sigmoid volvulus

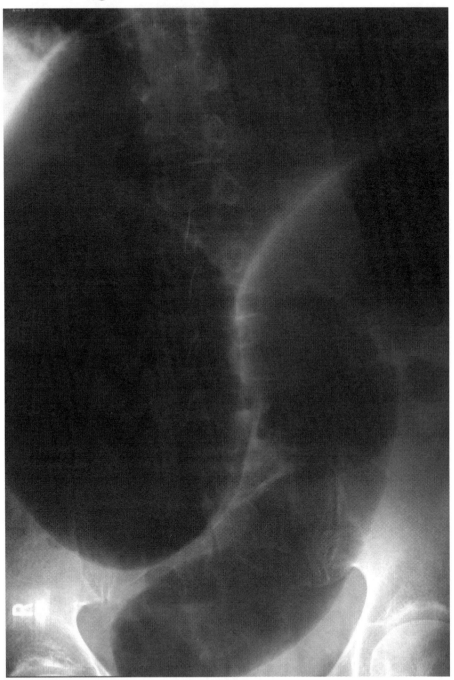

There is a hugely dilated loop of bowel extending from the pelvis with a characteristic inverted 'U' loop or 'coffee bean' appearance. These are the characteristic appearances of sigmoid volvulus.

## Background

Sigmoid volvulus classically results in a hugely dilated loop of bowel extending from the pelvis. The inverted 'U' loop or 'coffee bean' appearance is commonly devoid of haustra and is seen to extend as far as the liver in the right upper quadrant, and to the 10th thoracic vertebra superiorly. The inferior convergence of the two limbs of the loop is seen in the left iliac fossa. There may be some secondary loops of dilated large bowel associated with these appearances.

It is said that long-term inpatients in psychiatric institutions are particularly prone to the condition, possibly due to their medication or institutionalised diet.

## CASE 2.6 Caecal volvulus

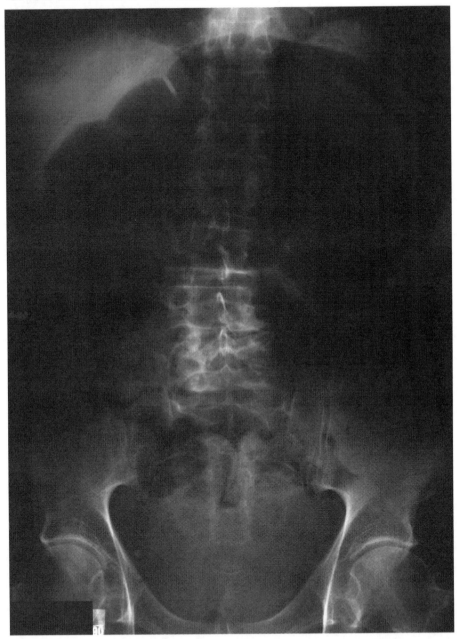

There is a markedly dilated air-filled viscus in the central abdomen. This is separate from the stomach, and does not appear to have the typical appearance of transverse colon, in that it does not extend from the expected positions of the hepatic and splenic flexures. Furthermore, the caecum is not present in the right iliac fossa. These appearances are therefore highly suspicious of caecal volvulus.

## Background

Caecal volvulus is far less common than sigmoid volvulus, since the caecum is usually a retroperitoneal structure. In some patients, however, the caecum hangs on a mesentery and is, therefore, at risk of twisting about its axis to lie across the midline in the upper/central abdomen. If the diameter of the caecum exceeds 9 cm there is risk of imminent perforation.

## CASE 2.7 Extraluminal gas

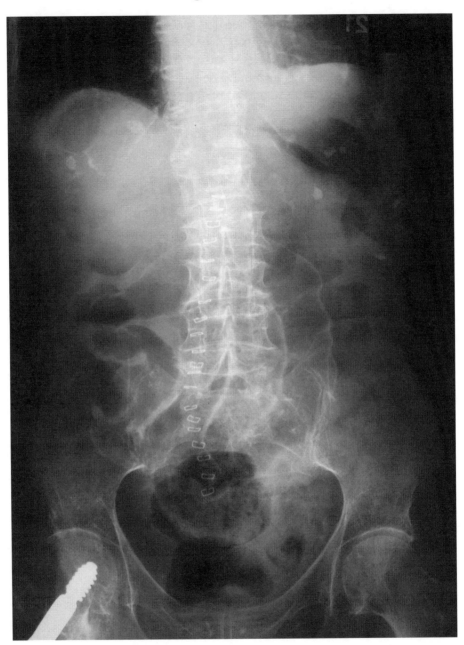

Supine abdominal radiograph showing clear definition of bowel loops, whereby both the mucosal and serosal surfaces are clearly seen. This is in keeping with free intraperitoneal gas. In this case, there are multiple metallic surgical clips suggesting recent laparotomy as the likely cause. If there is doubt as to the presence of free gas, an erect CXR should be performed (*Case 1.14*).

## Background

On the supine abdominal film, gas is normally only seen within the bowel lumen. This results in a clear inner margin of bowel due to air–mucosa interface. The outer margin (the serosal surface) however is not clearly seen since the serosal surfaces merge with those of adjacent loops. However, perforation results in free intraperitoneal gas forming an interface with the serosal surface, which then becomes radiographically visible, giving the appearance of a thin 'pencilled' line of the bowel wall with gas on either side. This appearance is known as Rigler's sign. On the supine film, peritoneal folds may also be outlined by gas, including the falciform ligament (*Figure 2.7a*) and the median, medial and lateral umbilical ligaments (peritoneal folds caused by the urachus, inferior epigastric vessels and obliterated umbilical arteries, respectively).

Free gas may be seen after bowel perforation, or following laparotomy or laparoscopy, or even following prolonged gastrointestinal endoscopy. In adults post-laparotomy pneumoperitoneum persists for up to 7 days, while in children it is often resorbed by 24 hours. Contrast studies may be used to diagnose an anastomotic leak or perforation. However, clinical correlation and CT is often indicated in these cases.

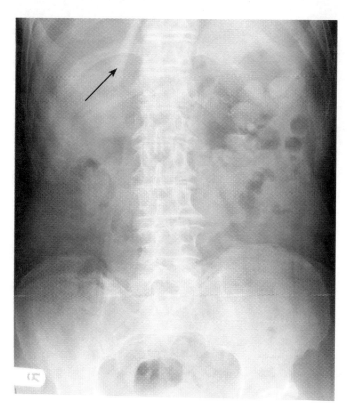

*Figure 2.7a. Air seen outlining the falciform ligament (arrow).*

## CASE 2.8 Abdominal aortic aneurysm

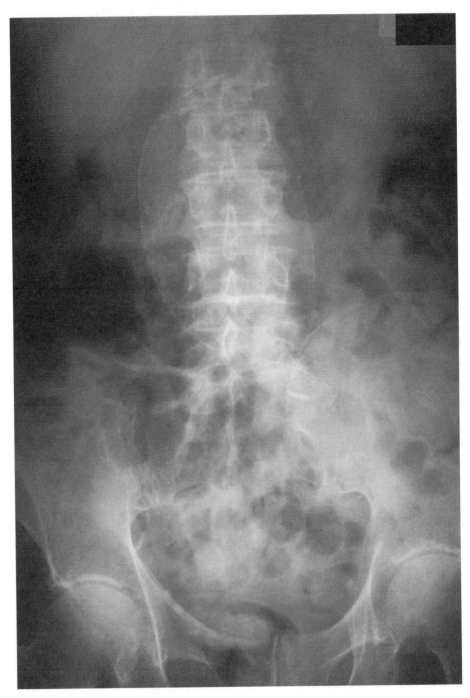

Supine abdominal radiograph showing characteristic appearance of a calcified fusiform aortic aneurysm.

## Background

The extent and shape of a calcified aortic aneurysm can be seen on a plain abdominal film. Rarely, loss of soft tissue planes adjacent to the psoas shadows may indicate retroperitoneal haemorrhage (*Figure 2.8a*). However, the psoas outlines may not be seen in the normal individual and therefore this is not a reliable indicator of retroperitoneal bleeding. The investigation of choice to exclude rupture in a stable patient is a contrast-enhanced CT scan of the abdomen (*Figure 2.8b*). If there is high suspicion of ruptured aortic aneurysm, the patient is often referred directly to theatre, particularly if there is evidence of cardiovascular compromise. Routine follow-up of aortic aneurysm size is usually by ultrasound. Other vascular structures commonly known to calcify include the iliac and splenic arteries (*Figure 2.8c*).

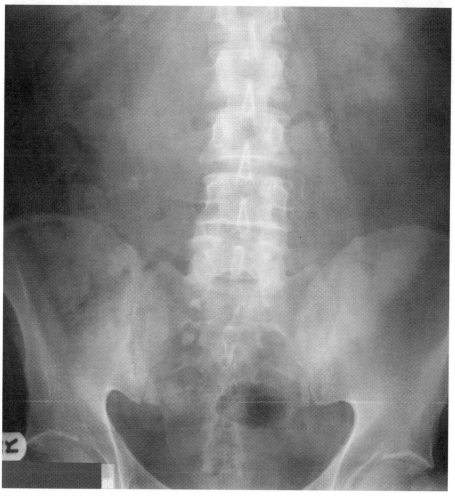

*Figure 2.8a. AXR with loss of fat plane adjacent to the psoas muscles. This may be a normal finding, but in this case was due to retroperitoneal haemorrhage. If there is suspicion of abdominal aortic aneurysm bleed, urgent CT and surgical referral is necessary.*

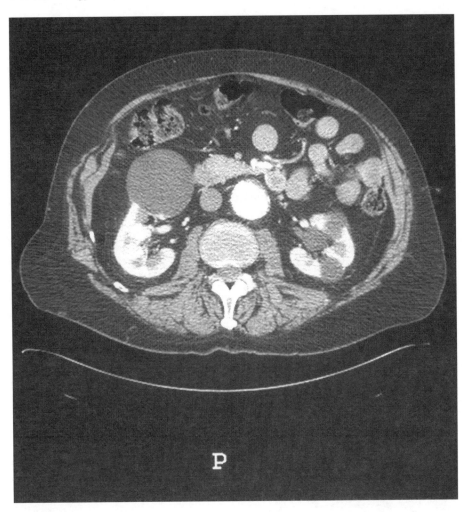

Figure 2.8b. Contrast-enhanced CT scan of the abdomen demonstrating an abdominal aortic aneurysm. Incidental renal cysts are also seen.

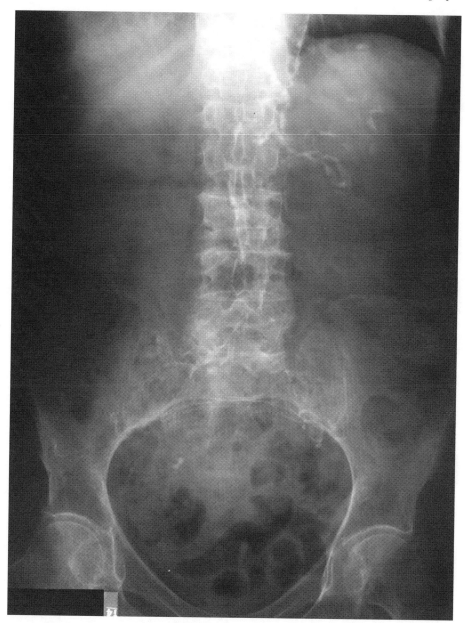

*Figure 2.8c. Plain abdominal radiograph showing typical serpiginous calcification in the left hypochondrium due to calcification within the wall of the splenic artery.*

## CASE 2.9 Calcified gallstones and renal stones

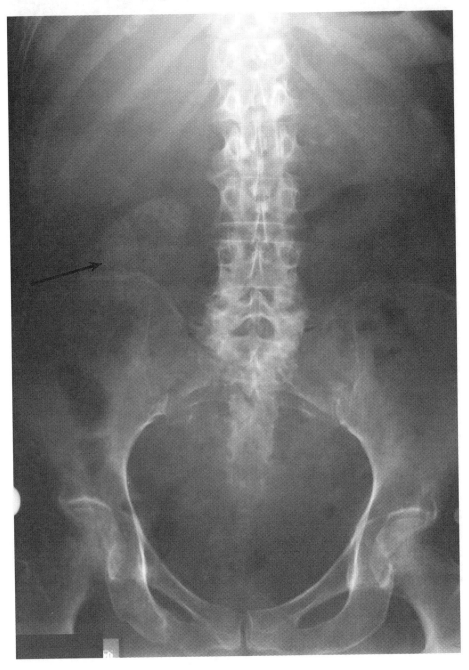

Calcified, multifaceted gallstones are seen on this image (arrow).

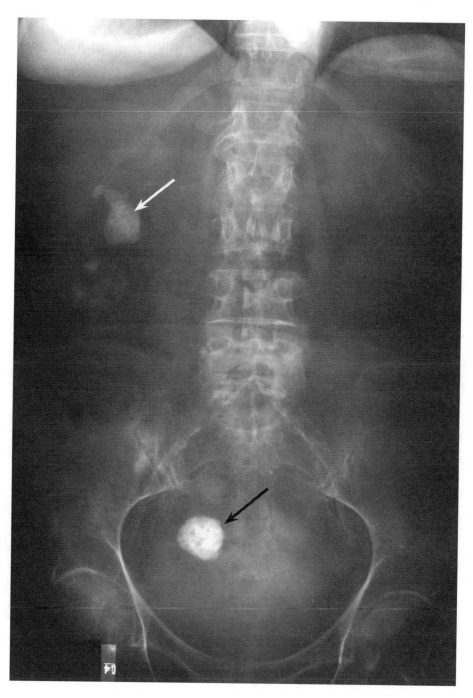

This shows staghorn renal calculus (white arrow). Also note whorled calcification within an incidental uterine fibroid (black arrow)

## Background

Abnormal calcification can be used to make a diagnosis in the following conditions:

- Gallstones (only 10% are radio-opaque) (See *Case 4.1*).
- Renal/ureteric/bladder stones (90% are radio-opaque) (See *Section 4*).
- Calcified lymphadenopathy (*Figure 2.9a*).
- Chronic pancreatitis (*Figure 2.9b*).
- Appendicolith (*Figure 2.9c*).
- Liver and spleen calcification – hepatomas, old abscesses, some metastases (*Figure 2.9d*).
- Uterine fibroids (appear as well-defined areas with whorled contents within the pelvis; they are usually an incidental finding).
- Adrenal gland calcification (usually due to previous TB).
- Prostate and seminal vesicle calcification (often incidental finding but occasionally due to previous TB).

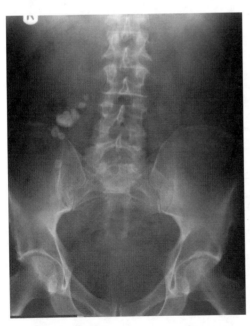 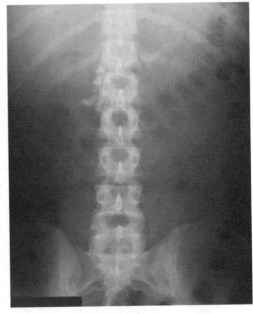

Figure 2.9a. Calcified lymphadenopathy – usually in the right iliac fossa due to previous tuberculosis in the lymph nodes adjacent to the terminal ileum.

Figure 2.9b. Calcification throughout the pancreas in keeping with chronic pancreatitis.

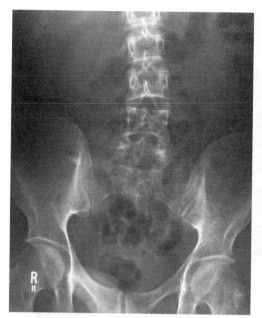

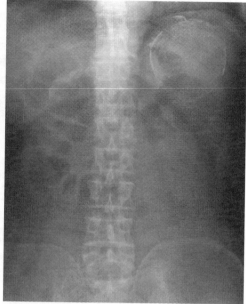

Figure 2.9c.. Calcified faecal appendicolith projected over the right iliac wing. When associated with right iliac fossa pain the diagnosis is appendicitis until proven otherwise.

Figure 2.9d. A large calcified cyst within the left upper quadrant suggesting long-standing splenic abscess probably due to hydatid disease.

## CASE 2.10 Ascites

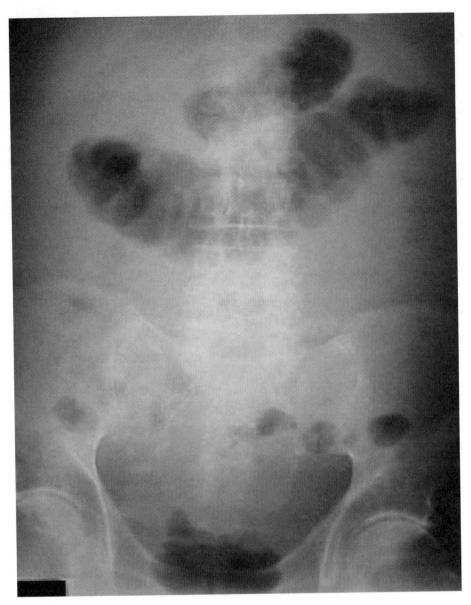

Plain abdominal radiograph showing uniform increased density extending across the abdomen, and particularly in both flanks. The gas-filled loops of bowel have floated into a central position and as a result there is a paucity of bowel in both flanks. These are the appearances of ascites.

## Background

The appearances of ascites on plain film are subtle. However, significant amounts of ascites tend to accumulate in the paracolic gutters and flanks, causing gas-filled loops of bowel to float towards the central abdomen, and the fluid appears as uniform soft tissue density across the abdomen. In addition, ascites within the pelvis may result in loss of the normal bladder outline. Ascites is usually confirmed on ultrasound scanning of the abdomen (*Figure 2.10a*).

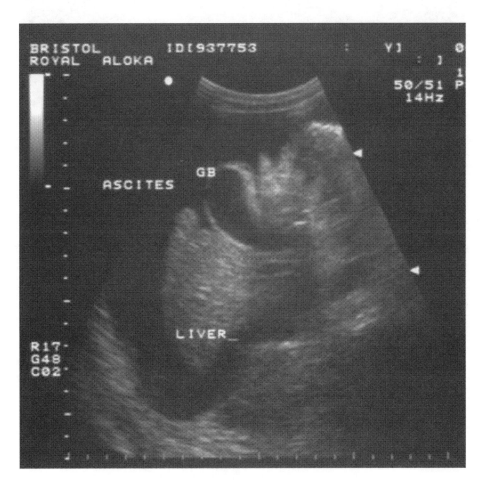

*Figure 2.10a. Ultrasound scan of the abdomen confirming a large amount of ascites.*

## CASE 2.11 Inguinal hernia

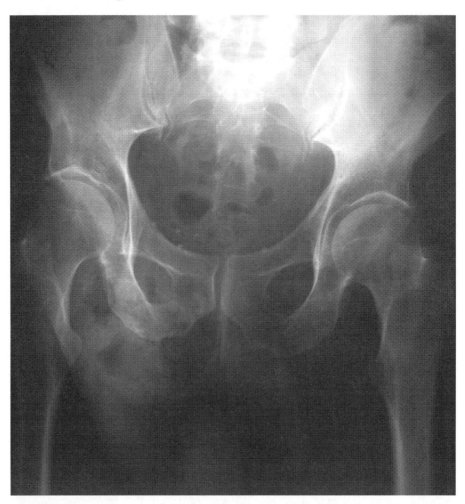

There is a large mass arising within the right iliac fossa, which appears to contain mixed density of soft tissue and gas. The appearances are in keeping with a large inguinal hernia containing sigmoid colon. There is no evidence of bowel obstruction.

## Background

Hernias are usually too small to be seen on plain radiography, but occasionally large hernias are apparent, when (as in this case) they contain loops of gas and faecal-laden bowel. Bowel is not usually seen below the line of the inguinal ligament (an imaginary line on the X-ray between the anterior superior iliac spine and the pubic tubercle as shown on *Figure 2.11a*). Occasionally, a true hernia can be difficult to distinguish from an apron of abdominal wall and bowel, as occurs in the obese patient with laxity of the musculature of the anterior abdominal wall. Hernias are a potential cause of bowel obstruction, or incarceration and ischaemia, as already mentioned (*Case 2.1*).

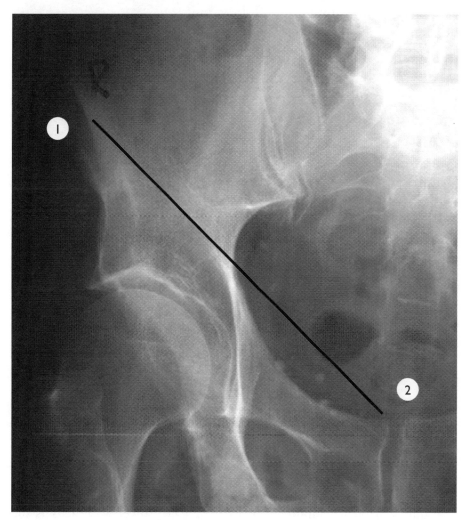

*Figure 2.11a. Plain AXR showing the line of the inguinal ligament between the anterior superior iliac spine (1) and the pubic tubercle (2).*

## CASE 2.12 Pneumatosis coli

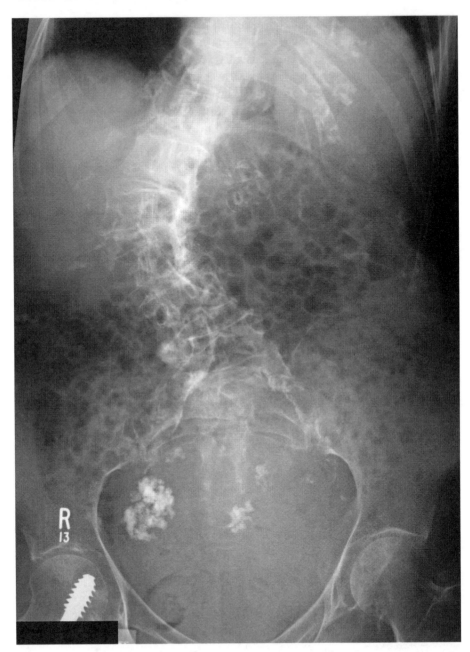

This is a supine abdominal radiograph showing the characteristic appearance of air-containing bubbles within the bowel wall. This is the typical appearance of pneumatosis coli. Note also the incidental presence of calcified uterine fibroids and iliac arteries within the pelvis, as well as a severe lumbar spine scoliosis.

## Background

Pneumatosis coli occurs as multiple small bubbles of gas within the bowel wall in a submucosal position. It is seen in association with obstructive airways disease but the mechanism of this association is not clear. Occasionally, a gas-filled bleb may rupture and result in a benign cause of free intraperitoneal gas.

## CASE 2.13 Soft tissue mass

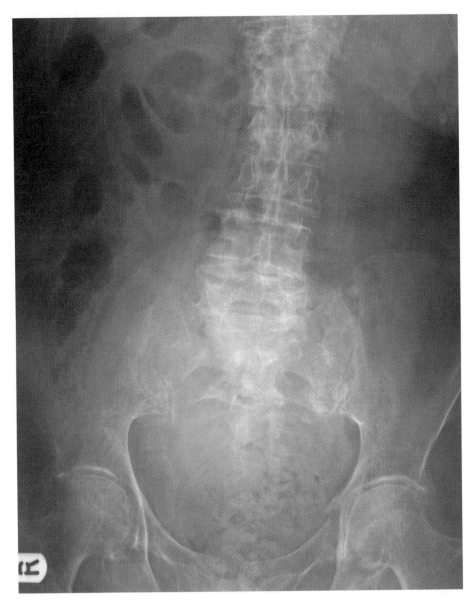

There is a mass arising within the pelvis, which is causing displacement of the adjacent loops of bowel. This is likely to represent either ovarian tumour or enlarged bladder. An ultrasound scan would be appropriate to further evaluate this

## Background

The outlines of the liver and spleen may be seen as soft tissue outlines displacing loops of bowel from the right and left upper quadrants, respectively. The renal outlines may also be seen in their retroperitoneal position outlined by fat (note that due to their retroperitoneal position that renal enlargement will not usually cause bowel displacement). Within the pelvis, the bladder may also be seen as a uniform area of fluid or soft tissue density, and a pelvic tumour may mimic this, and cause displacement of bowel superiorly.

If an apparent soft tissue mass is seen to contain bubbles of gas (*Figure 2.13a*), then this is likely to either represent an abscess containing gas-forming organisms, or indicate a fistulous connection with bowel.

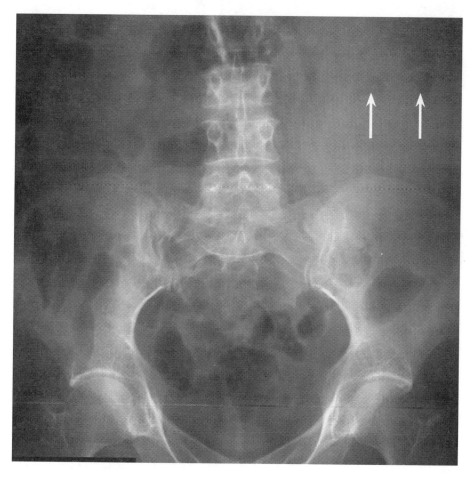

*Figure 2.13a. There is a soft tissue mass on the left side of the abdomen, which contains several bubbles of gas within it (arrows). This is not typical for bowel gas, and the appearances are most likely to be due to intra-abdominal abscess (this would have to be correlated with the clinical findings). Ultrasound or CT scans would be appropriate to further evaluate this.*

## CASE 2.14 Barium studies

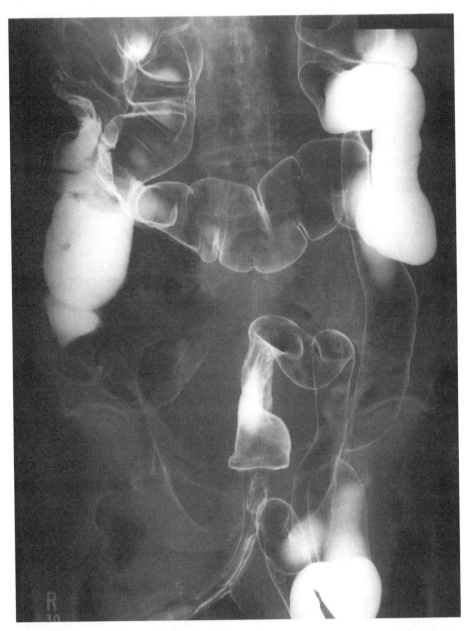

A double-contrast film from a barium enema series with contrast seen extending as far as the caecal pole. There are bilateral inguinal hernias; that on the left contains sigmoid colon, but the right-sided hernia contains only gas and must therefore contain small bowel.

## Background

Contrast examinations of the gastrointestinal tract include:

* barium swallow for examination of the oesophagus
* barium meal for examination of the stomach
* barium follow-through for examination of the small bowel
* barium enema for examination of the colon.

The barium swallow and barium meal examinations have been largely replaced by the use of endoscopy, but are still performed in some cases if the patient will not tolerate endoscopic examinations, or for evaluation of dysmotility disorders that would not be appreciated by endoscopy. Endoscopy has the advantage of being able to take biopsies of any suspicious area to confirm the diagnosis (eg. gastric malignancy).

Barium follow-through examinations are still commonly performed because of the inability of an endoscope to easily reach this part of the gastrointestinal tract. Follow-through examinations are either performed by asking the patient to swallow a quantity of barium, then performing a series of abdominal radiographs and screening as the contrast passes through the small bowel, or occasionally by passing a naso-enteral tube to fill and distend the small bowel directly.

Barium enema examinations are also still widely performed, commonly for changes in bowel habit or lower gastrointestinal bleeding. As with barium examinations of the upper gastrointestinal tract, the barium enema is unable to give a histologically proven diagnosis, and so colonoscopy may still be required. However, barium enema is readily available, clearly depicts colonic tumours (*Figure 2.14a*), and has a lower complication rate than colonoscopy. Barium enema is also better at visualising the entirety of the colon since the colonoscope may not reach the caecal pole in all cases.

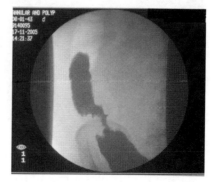

*Figure 2.14a. Single film from barium enema demonstrating classical 'apple core' abnormality in keeping with primary colonic carcinoma.*

## CASE 2.15 Abdominal foriegn bodies

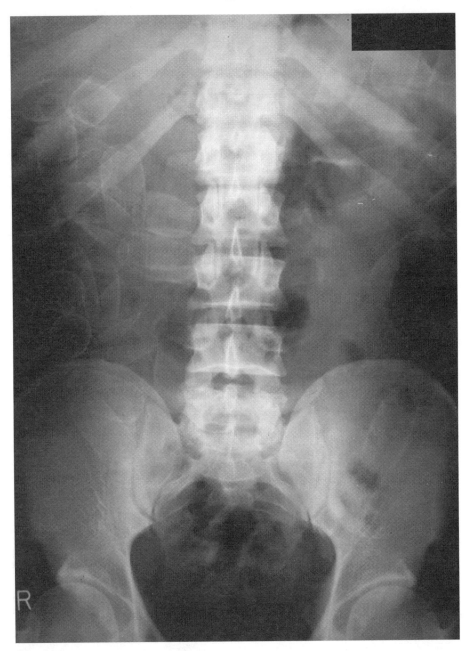

AXR showing multiple lozenge-shaped densities throughout the abdomen, which do not conform to any natural anatomical structure. They are likely to represent drug-filled condoms, a technique used for the illegal transportation of illicit drugs by a so-called 'drug mule'.

## Background

We are all taught to diagnose pathology, but may forget to consider patient-related abnormal appearances such as that seen here. Other appearances might include that seen in *Figure 2.15a*. When faced with such bizarre appearances always ensure that these are not due to densities or objects on the patient's clothing or skin surface.

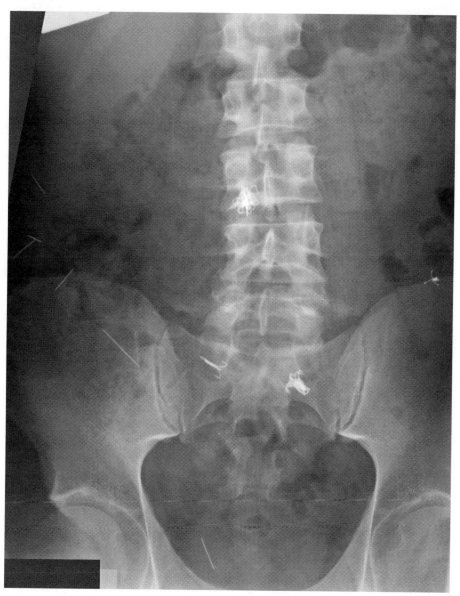

Figure 2.15a. Plain AXR showing multiple metallic densities within the abdomen due to the ingestion of needles and fish hooks by a psychiatric patient.

# Section 3

# Musculoskeletal Radiology

# Introduction

Plain radiographs are the mainstay of evaluating the skeleton, both in the evaluation of trauma, and in the diagnosis and follow-up of other bone pathologies including primary bone tumours, metastatic disease, multiple myeloma, and the arthritides. This section is not a definitive orthopaedic or rheumatological text, but it reviews the appearances of commonly occuring bone pathology that may be encountered in medical or surgical examinations.

This introduction is divided into two parts, first, non-traumatic bone and joint pathology and, second, trauma with a selection of commonly encountered fractures.

### *Non-traumatic bone and joint pathology: basic principles*

In assessing a plain film for evidence of musculoskeletal disease, remember to evaluate the soft tissues as well as the underlying bone. As we shall see, this is particularly important in the evaluation of trauma when soft tissue injury, foreign bodies or joint effusions may be seen on the film. However, review of the soft tissues for oedema, haematoma, or inflammatory change is equally important in cases of non-traumatic bone or joint pathology.

After review of the soft tissues, the bones must be evaluated. Differentiation must be made between primary bone and joint pathology. This is done by evaluating whether the area of abnormality appears to be centred on a joint (ie. involving both sides of a joint space) or occurs within the bone. The most common arthritides are rheumatoid arthritis and degenerative osteoarthritis, and these are discussed in detail in *Cases 3.8* and *3.9*, respectively.

As we shall see in *Cases 3.2–3.4*, the terms sclerosis and lysis must also be understood. An area of *sclerosis* is said to occur if the bone is of increased density, and *lysis* is the converse.

If a lesion has been identified within a bone it should also be possible to ascertain if this is likely to be an aggressive or benign lesion. This differentiation is probably best done by assessing the zone of transition between the abnormal lesion and the adjacent normal bone. A narrow, well-defined *zone of transition* is likely to represent a benign lesion since the pathological process has not infiltrated into the adjacent bone. This is discussed further on p. 127. Aggressive lesions are usually due to malignancy (primary bone tumours or secondary bone metastases) or due to infective changes (osteomyelitis).

### *Trauma: basic principles*

After clinical examination, the plain radiograph is of the utmost importance to determine if a fracture has occurred. Fractures may be obvious (*Figure 3A*), but other less obvious patterns of bone injury may be present. Fractures are classically seen as an irregular, non-corticated line traversing the bone. There may be associated soft tissue swelling due to haematoma or joint effusion.

Fracture lines should not be confused with the smooth, well-demarcated, and often branching appearance of intraosseous blood vessels. Similarly, ensure a potential fracture line is indeed limited to the bone, and does not extend into the adjacent soft tissues, which will occur if it is actually due to an overlying soft tissue shadow.

Trauma should always be imaged by two films, usually taken at approximately $90^0$ to each other (ie. a frontal view and a lateral projection). This is because a subtle fracture may not be seen on a single projection, but more importantly even significantly displaced fractures or dislocations may not be apparent on a single film if the pathology is in the same plane as the projection of the film (*Figure 3B*).

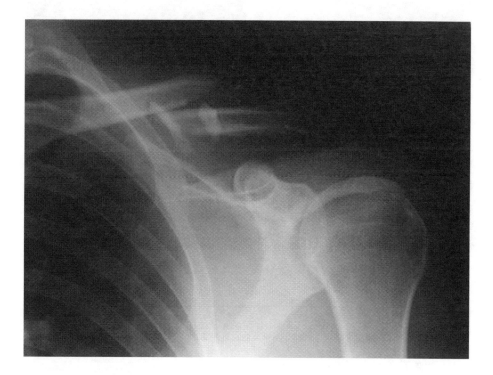

*Figure 3A. Comminuted fracture to the left clavicle.*

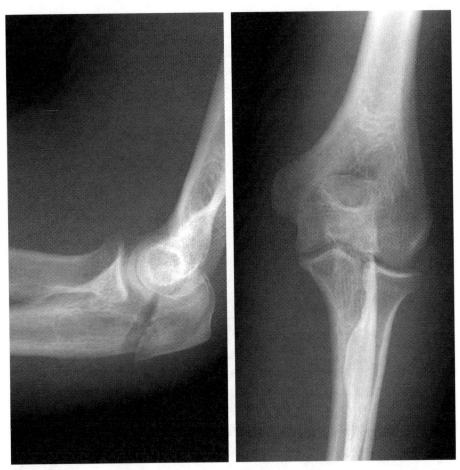

Figure 3B. Fractured olecranon visible on lateral projection but not readily apparent on the AP projection.

---

**Key points of musculoskeletal radiology**

- Always assess soft tissues as well as bone.
- Determine if a bone abnormality is related to a joint (ie. representing a joint pathology) or is arising within the bone distinct from a joint.
- Know and understand the terms *sclerosis* and *lysis*.
- Understand the term *zone of transition* and its use in determining between aggressive and non-aggressive bone lesions.
- Two films in different planes are usually needed to exclude fracture or dislocations.

# Fracture types of particular interest

Before looking at *Cases 3.1–2.9,* here is a series of commonly occuring bone pathologies you might come across during medical or surgical examinations.

## *Colle's fracture*

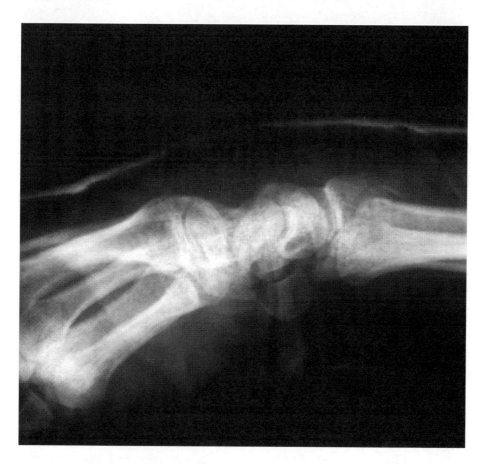

There is a fracture to the distal radius with dorsal (backward) tilt and dorsal angulation. These are the appearances of a Colle's fracture. This fracture has already been immobilised in a plaster cast.

Colle's fracture has come to mean a fracture within the distal 2.5 cm of the lower radius, with backward tilt and displacement. The distal fragment may be displaced radially. This fracture typically occurs as a result of falling on the outstretched arm, and results in the 'dinner fork' deformity. Its classical appearances should be differentiated from a Smith's fracture whereby the fracture results in dorsal angulation and palmar displacement. Smith's fractures occur typically in motorcycle trauma because the hand is often not extended on impact.

### Radial head fracture

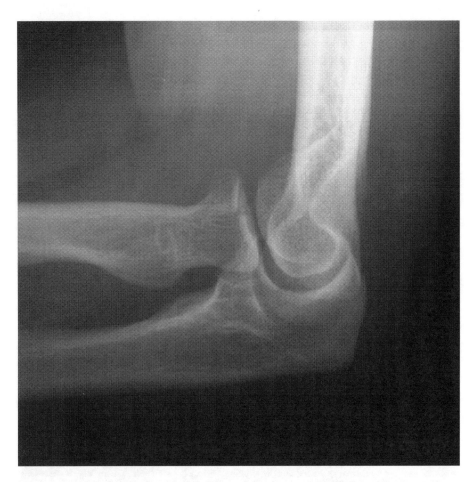

There is a radial head fracture extending towards the radial neck. There is a large joint effusion manifested by anterior and posterior fat pad signs. Radial head fractures are not always visible on the initial plain film. However, the presence of a displaced fat pad suggests the presence of a joint effusion, and thus a probable underlying fracture.

*The fat pad sign:* the anterior fat pad may be just visible in normal cases as a narrow triangle anterior to the distal humerus, but when this is enlarged, or if any posterior pad is seen, this constitutes fat pad displacement which is likely to indicate joint effusion and thus underlying radial head fracture. In the paediatric age group a supra-condylar fracture to the distal humerus may also give rise to the fat pad sign.

## Lipohaemarthrosis

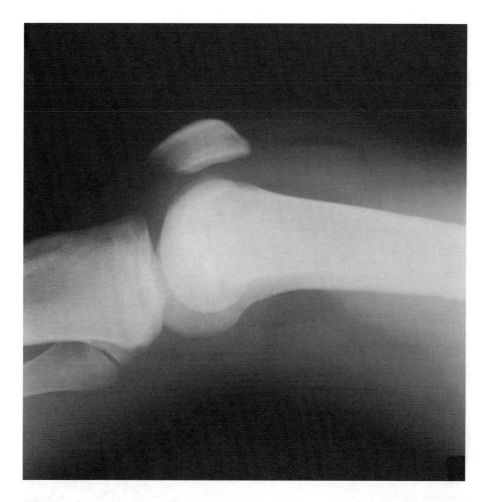

There is a lipohaemarthrosis of the knee joint. This is the presence of blood and fat (from bone marrow) within the joint space, and indicates the presence of underlying tibial plateau fracture. The film is best viewed horizontally, as shown here to demonstrate the lipohaemarthrosis as a fluid level.

## Scaphoid fracture

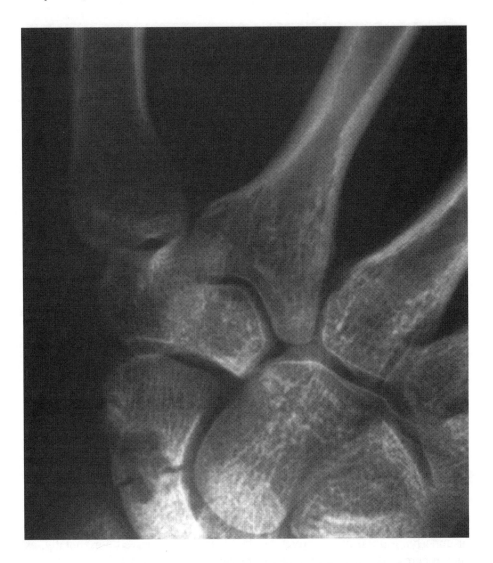

There is a fracture through the waist of the scaphoid. These fractures are particularly noteworthy because if they are not diagnosed and immobilised they may result in avascular necrosis. Avascular necrosis affects the proximal segment since the blood flow occurs to this area from the distal part of the bone; the fracture will transect intraosseus and periosteal vessels resulting in necrosis. Necrosis will result in sclerosis, and possible fragmentation. This image shows avascular necrosis of the proximal scaphoid, with the fracture line still evident.

## Neck of femur fracture

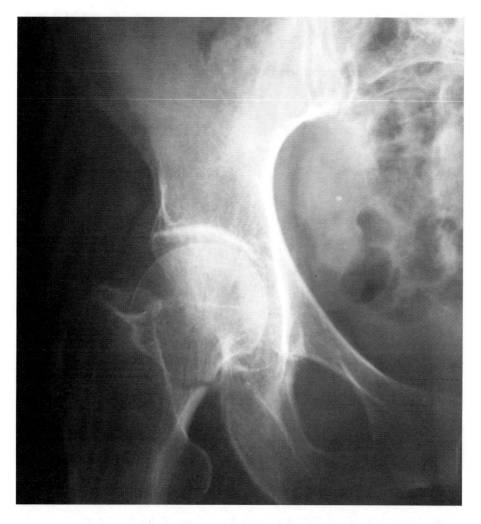

There is a subcapital fracture to the neck of femur (NOF). Fractures to the NOF may be classified as follows:

* subcapital
* transcervical
* intertrochanteric (actually extracapsular and therefore not strictly an NOF fracture).

The subcapital intracapsular fracture is particularly noteworthy. This is because the blood supply to the femoral head largely reaches it via the femoral neck. A subcapital fracture is therefore most likely to interrupt this blood supply, and thus may impede healing and ultimately result in ischaemic necrosis to the femoral head.

## CASE 3.1 Paget's disease

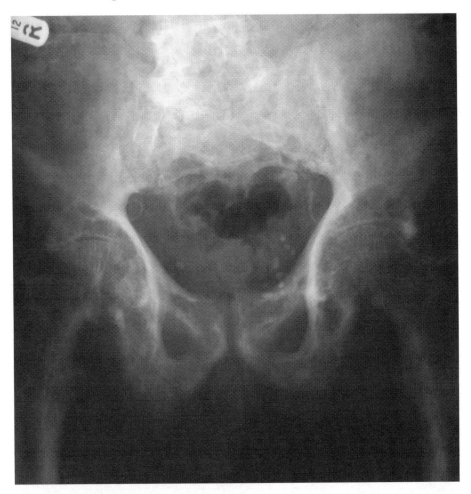

There is thickening of the bone cortex, with associated coarsening of the trabecular pattern, and overall bone expansion. These appearances are seen throughout the bones of the pelvis and proximal femora, and are typical of Paget's disease.

## Background

Paget's disease of bone occurs in the elderly population, and is usually asymptomatic. It is a disease of abnormal bone turnover and modelling, resulting in thickening of the bone cortex, coarsening of the trabecular pattern, and overall bone expansion. The disease typically affects the bones of the pelvis, spine, skull, and proximal long bones but can affect any bone. It is, however, only very rarely seen in the fibula or mandible. Paget's can rarely (1%) be complicated by the development of a malignant osteogenic sarcoma. These tumours are classically lytic, and originate within the femora as a poorly defined area of bone destruction. Paget's disease is also clearly seen on CT scan (*Figure 3.1a*).

*Look-alikes*: The appearances of Paget's disease can be confused with the diffuse sclerotic metastases seen in carcinoma of the prostate gland. However, these pathologies may be differentiated by lack of trabecular thickening and expansion in sclerotic metastases, which often also result in foci of sclerosis rather than the more uniform pattern seen in Paget's. In clinical practice, if doubt persists, then these pathologies may be discriminated by measurement of the plasma prostate-specific antigen (PSA) level.

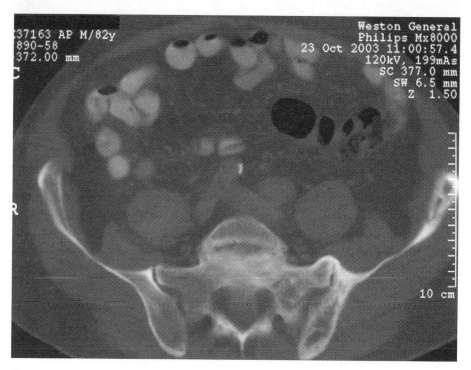

Figure 3.1a. CT scan of the pelvis showing coarsening and expansion of the left iliac wing (different patient from Case 3.1).

## CASE 3.2 Sclerotic bone metastases

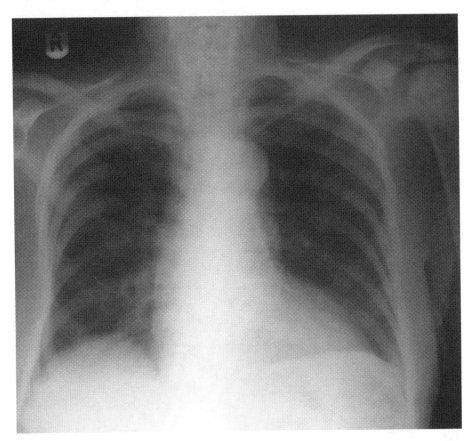

There is evidence of widespread sclerosis affecting all of the ribs, with further involvement of the clavicles, scapulae and proximal humeri. These are the appearances of diffuse sclerotic bone metastases most usually seen in carcinoma of the prostate.

## Background

Also note in *Case 3.2* there is evidence of breast tissue shadows (particularly on the left side). These represent areas of abnormal breast tissue formation (gynaecomastia) in the male sex, which would have occurred in this case if the patient had been subjected to hormonal treatment (anti-androgenic) for his prostatic primary.

Sclerotic metastases typically occur from potential primary malignancies of the prostate, breast, stomach and carcinoid. Therefore, if there are appearances that suggest diffuse sclerotic bone metastases in a female patient, look for evidence of breast asymmetry or mastectomy which would be confirmatory of breast surgery for primary malignancy.

The diffuse bone sclerosis seen in cases of metastases is not always readily apparent because inexperienced observers often assume the appearances relate to features of the radiograph itself, rather than diffuse pathology (*Figure 3.2a*).

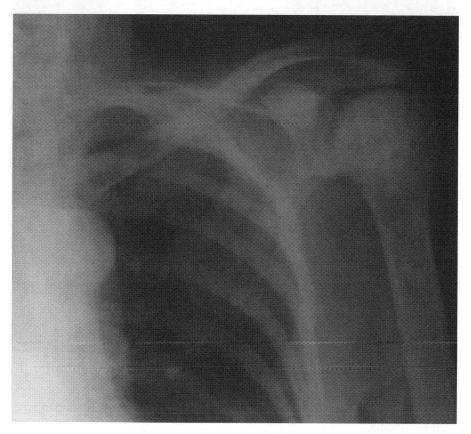

*Figure 3.2a. Confluent areas of sclerosis in keeping with prostatic metastases.*

## CASE 3.3 Lytic bone metastases

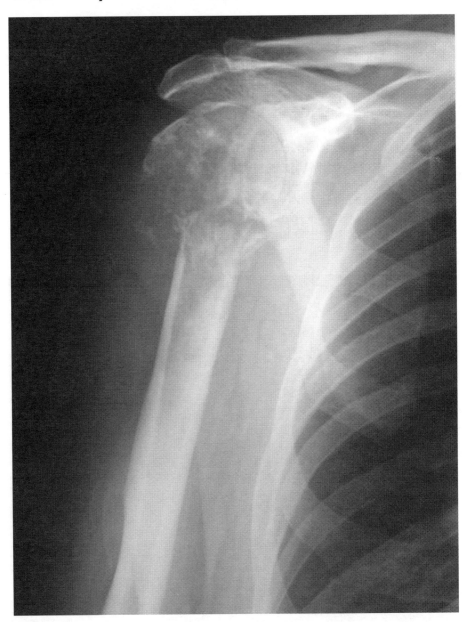

There is an area of poorly defined bone destruction involving the entire right humeral head. These are the appearances of lytic bone metastasis due to renal cell carcinoma.

## Background

Bone metastases resulting in lysis (bone destruction) occur due to metastatic disease from the following primary malignancies:

* lung
* breast (more usually causes sclerosis)
* kidney
* thyroid
* bladder.

As in all cases, review of the radiograph may give clues as to the actual primary in any one case. For example, on a chest radiograph the lung primary may be seen, or there may be evidence of a superior mediastinal mass due to thyroid primary. Alternatively, there may be evidence of surgery performed in the treatment of the patient's primary malignancy (see *Figure 3.3a*).

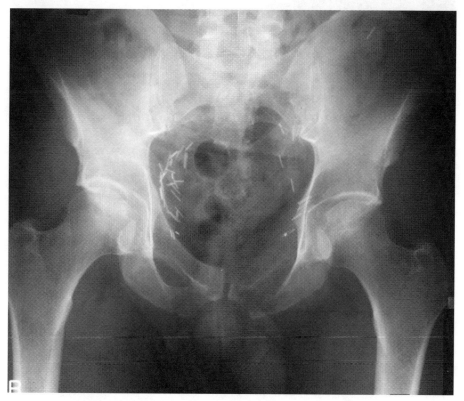

*Figure 3.3a. X-ray of the pelvis showing lytic destruction of the left superior pubic ramus in keeping with bone metastasis. Note should be made of the metallic surgical clips within the pelvis. This patient has undergone cystectomy in the treatment of transitional cell carcinoma of the bladder.*

## CASE 3.4 Multiple myeloma

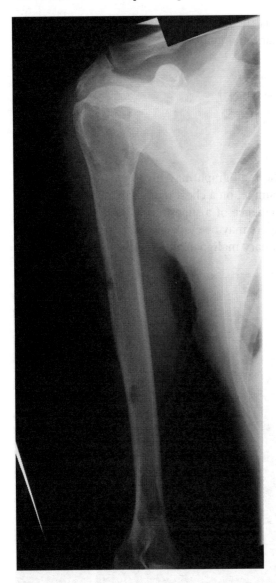

There are multiple well-defined lytic lesions within the right humerus, with endosteal scalloping, and a narrow zone of transition suggesting these are not overtly aggressive. Furthermore, subtle lesions are seen within several of the ribs, and at least one probable pathological fracture is seen through one of these areas. These appearances are in keeping with multiple myeloma.

In the second image, the pathological fracture is indicated by an arrow.

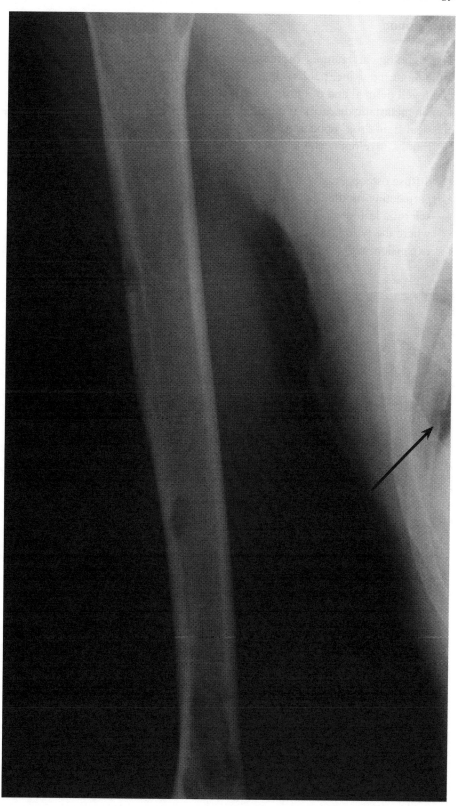

## Background

The radiological features of multiple myeloma include multiple lucencies throughout the spine, pelvis, skull, ribs, and shafts of long bones. These are often well defined and of uniform size (compared with the varying sizes often seen in metastatic disease). Where these occur in the skull, they give rise to the classical 'rain drop' appearance (see *Figure 3.4a*).

Rarely, myeloma can cause any of the following:

* diffuse osteopaenia
* permeating mottled appearances due to more aggressive bone destruction
* sclerotic lesions (2–3% of cases)
* where the lytic lesions affect the ribs, there may be evidence of expansion with associated soft tissue masses (*Figure 3.4c*).

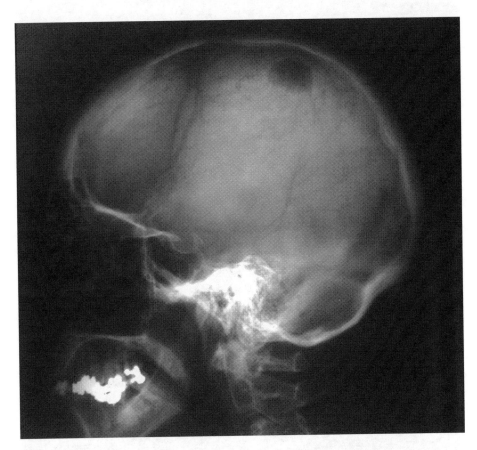

*Figure 3.4b. Single moderate-sized lucency to the skull vault giving the classical appearance of a myeloma deposit. Note this lesion is larger than those seen in hyperparathyroidism ('pepper pot' skull).*

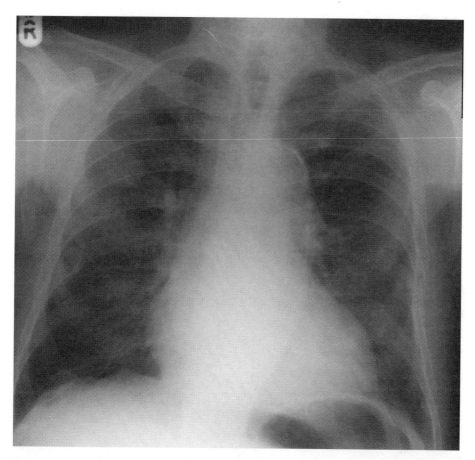

*Figure 3.4c. Lucencies to the right lower ribs, with associated soft tissue expansion, in keeping with myeloma.*

## Zone of transition

The zone of transition is invaluable in assessing whether a lesion is likely to be benign or aggressive (malignant or infective) in cause. The zone of transition is the line that demarcates normal from abnormal bone. If the transition is well defined, and normal bone can be easily discriminated from adjacent abnormal bone (eg. a pencil line can be drawn between the two) then this is said to be a narrow zone and it is likely to be due to benign pathology. If, on the other hand, the zone of transition is wide, then this is likely to be due to aggressive pathology such as malignancy or infection.

127

## CASE 3.5 Osteopaenia

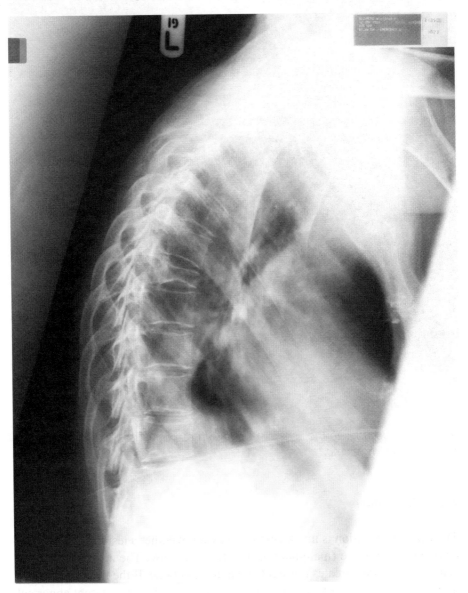

In this lateral radiograph of the thoracic and upper lumbar spine there is an overall loss of bone density, with particular thinning of the cortex, and relative prominence of the primary trabecular pattern. In addition there is a compression fracture at approximately the T6 level.

## Background

These are the typical appearances of osteopaenia in an elderly person. Remember that almost identical appearances to osteoporosis are seen in cases of osteomalacia and rickets. For this reason the term osteopaenia is commonly used in radiological reports, because it draws attention purely to the end result of bone loss, rather than the underlying cause. The causes of these appearances are listed here:

- Osteoporosis:
  - disuse
  - old age
  - Cushing syndrome
  - diabetes
  - drugs (eg. steroids, heparin)
  - deficiency states such as vitamin C (scurvy) or protein-energy malnutrition.
- Osteomalacia and rickets:
  - vitamin D deficiency (dietary, malabsorption, or behavioural – shielded from sun by clothing)
  - renal disease
  - hepatic disease
  - drugs (eg. phenytoin).

## CASE 3.6 Hyperparathyroidism

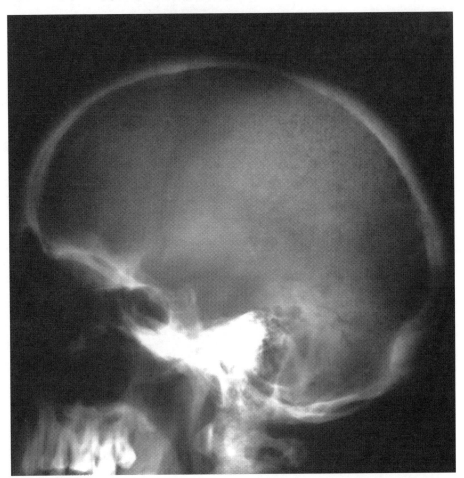

There are multiple small lucencies seen throughout the calvarium, which are smaller than those seen in myeloma or metastatic disease. These appearances are most likely to represent the diffuse changes of hyperparathyroidism causing the so-called 'pepper pot' skull appearance.

## Background

Hyperparathyroidism can occur due to any of the following:

- *Primary hyperparathyroidism:* adenoma, diffuse hyperplasia, adrenal carcinoma, or ectopic production of parathyroid hormone (PTH) from, for example, carcinoma of the bronchus.
- *Secondary to renal failure* in an attempt to restore the calcium/phosphate balance that occurs in renal disease.
- *Tertiary hyperparathyroidism*: this may occur in cases of pre-existing secondary hyperparathyroidism. It occurs if an adenoma over-develops and ultimately over-compensates for the renal-induced inbalance.

The radiological appearances include the following:

- *Pepper pot skull*
- *Subperiosteal bone resorption*
    - radial side of phalanges of middle and ring fingers (*Figure 3.6a*)
    - lateral end of clavicle
    - medial side of the proximal tibia
    - femoral neck (giving 'rotting fence-post' appearance).
- *Brown tumour*: a solitary lucency (eg. pelvis, tibia or femur) (*Figure 3.6b*) that occurs due to haemoglobin degradation products focally deposited within the bone.
- *Osteoacrolysis*: literally meaning lysis of the bone ends/high points ('acropolis' being the highest part of the city); this usually causes tapering of the terminal phalanges (*Figure 3.6a*).
- *Soft-tissue calcification and vascular calcification*: in the soft tissues, this typically occurs in cartilage, causing chondrocalcinosis.

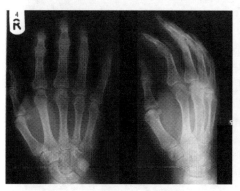

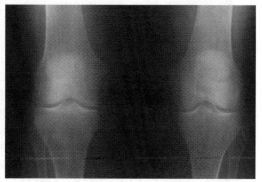

Figure 3.6a. There is lucency to the radial side of the phalanges of the middle and ring fingers in keeping with subperiosteal bone resorption. There is also tapering of the terminal phalanges in keeping with osteoacrolysis, and vascular calcification at the wrist. This patient had secondary hyperparathyroidism due to renal failure.

Fig.ure 3.6b. Lucency in the proximal right tibia in keeping with a brown tumour

## CASE 3.7 Ankylosing spondylitis

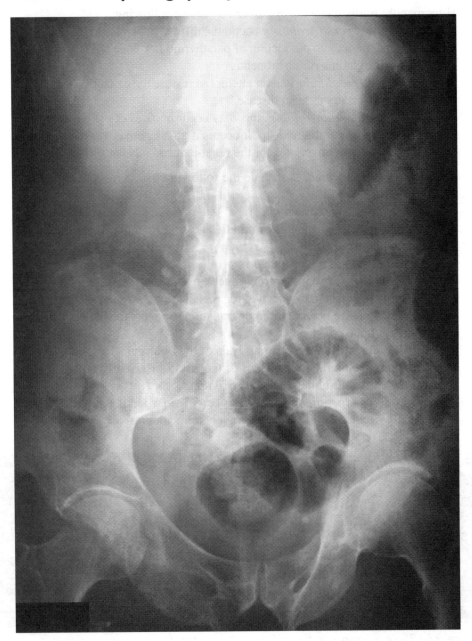

There is ankylosis of the lumbar vertebral bodies, and evidence of interspinous ligament calcification. The sacroiliac joints also appear fused with particular involvement of the left side. Note the incidental changes of Paget's disease in the right inferior pubic ramus.

## Background

Ankylosing spondylitis classically gives rise to low back pain in young adult males, with progression over time. It is associated with the HLA B27 haplotype in over 96% of cases.

The disease process usually begins with ankylosis of the sacroiliac joints, with progressive ankylosis of the lumbar and thoracolumbar spines to give the classical 'bamboo' spine appearance. The entirety of the spine can ultimately be affected. Due to the resultant ankylosis, with increasingly poor mobility and resultant disuse osteopaenia, these patients are predisposed to fracture (*Figure 3.7a*).

In addition, the costotransverse, costovertebral and posterior interspinous ligaments calcify, and there may be asymmetrical arthritic changes to the hips and shoulders, giving a similar appearance to rheumatoid arthritis.

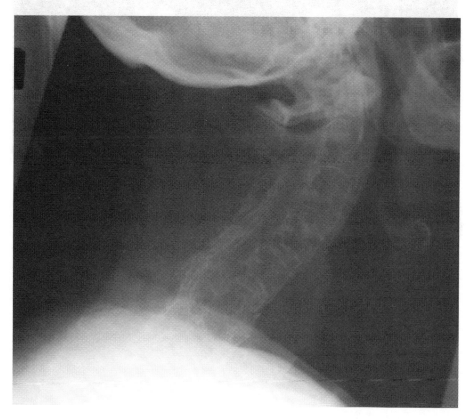

*Figure 3.7a. Complete ankylosis of the entire cervical spine, with some sparing at C1–2 level (where there is now excessive degenerative sclerosis due to this being the sole level of retained mobility). There is a fracture of the C6 vertebral body. The interspinous ligaments are splayed at this level, suggesting that the injury is unstable.*

## CASE 3.8 Rheumatoid arthritis

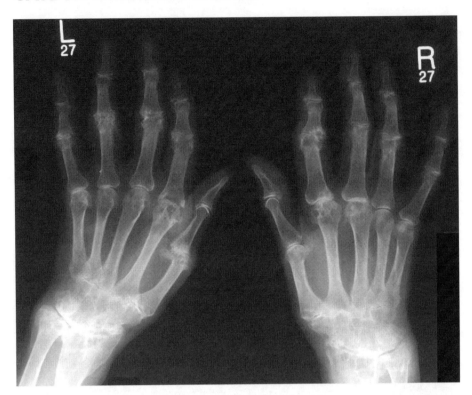

There is bilateral symmetrical erosive arthritis involving the metacarpal phalangeal joints. There is periarticular osteopaenia, and angulation of these joints (resulting in the classical 'swan neck' and 'Z-thumb' deformities). There is almost complete ankylosis of the carpus, and there is associated erosion of the ulnar styloid.

## Background

Rheumatoid arthritis is a multisystem disorder resulting in a symmetrical arthritis, most commonly affecting the hands, feet, ankles and elbows. The joints classically involved in the hand are the metacarpophalangeal and the proximal interphalangeal joints.

Rheumatoid arthritis is manifested by the following:

* synovial inflammation giving *soft tissue swelling*
* hyperaemia and disuse due to pain causing *periarticular osteopaenia*
* pannus growth resulting in *periarticular erosions* and *subchondral cysts*
* capsular and ligamentous laxity causing *deformity*
* *bone ankylosis.*

In longstanding cases involving the weight-bearing joints, there may be *secondary degenerative changes.*

## CASE 3.9 Degenerative osteoarthritis

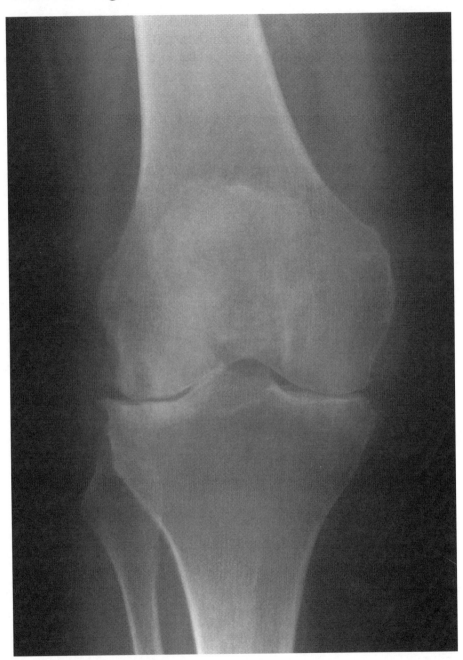

This plain film of the right knee reveals loss of joint space, subchondral sclerosis, and lateral osteophyte formation. In addition there is a single subchondral cyst in the distal lateral femoral condyle. These appearances are in keeping with degenerative osteoarthritis.

### Background

Degenerative osteoarthritis is manifested by the following:

* joint-space narrowing
* subchondral sclerosis
* subchondral cysts
* osteophyte formation
* relative preservation of bone density (cf. rheumatoid arthritis).

# Section 4

# Intravenous Urography and Imaging of the Urinary Tract

## Introduction

There are a number of techniques available in the evaluation of the urinary tract, including plain radiography, the intravenous urogram (IVU), ultrasound, and computed tomography. Recently, magnetic resonance imaging has also been used. These modalities will be discussed in turn. However, the IVU is the most widely available imaging technique and one of the first-line investigations, and therefore deserves a whole section of its own.

### Imaging of the renal tract

The simplest imaging modality remains the *plain radiograph* of the abdomen which has been localised (coned) to the area of the urinary tract in order to reduce exposure to the peripheral soft tissues. This examination is thus referred to as the *KUB (kidneys, ureters, bladder)*. The KUB is widely used as a first-line investigation of the urological tract, predominantly in the diagnosis of calcified (and therefore radio-opaque) stones. This simple investigation will detect 90% of such calculi, but evaluation can be difficult if there are large quantities of bowel gas or calcified costochondral cartilages, which may obscure small calculi. Similarly, calcified pelvic phleboliths (calcification within the walls of perivesical veins) can be confused for calculi at the vesicoureteric orifices. Phleboliths may be discriminated by their round smooth outlines, and sometimes a central lucency corresponding to the vein lumen. Consequently, an IVU may be needed to confirm this distinction. The KUB may also demonstrate the renal outlines although, as described below, the renal parenchyma is better seen on US. Despite its limitations the KUB remains an important initial examination, particularly for urinary tract calculi.

The intravenous urogram (IVU), as mentioned before, is another commonly used investigation. The IVU aids in the diagnosis of many urinary tract pathologies, including calculi, malignancy, obstruction and anatomical variants. The IVU is discussed in detail below.

Ultrasound (US) has a very important role in renal tract imaging. It is excellent in evaluating the soft tissues of the renal parenchyma. In addition, US is used to diagnose renal obstruction which is manifested by a dilated renal collecting system referred to as hydronephrosis (see Case 5.2). US is not commonly used in the evaluation of the ureter but may be used in the evaluation of the bladder, both for bladder volumes and prostate size, as well as the detection of bladder tumours. Bladder tumours are usually subsequently confirmed by cystoscopy.

The use of computed tomography (CT) has increased as it has become more widely available. CT may be used for detailed analysis of small intraparenchymal lesions, as well as for the staging of renal tumours.

*Computed tomography* KUB (CT KUB) is used increasingly in the investigation of renal colic due to stone disease. This technique involves performing a fine-slice, non-contrast-enhanced scan from the kidneys to the pubic symphysis. Due to the absence of contrast this will identify calculi, but will also indicate whether the upper tracts are obstructed, as well as further evaluating perirenal and other intra-abdominal pathology. It has the advantage of not using intravenous water-soluble contrast media, and thus avoids the risks associated with them. It is also rapidly performed, but involves a slightly higher radiation dose than the IVU (see *Case 5.13*).

*Magnetic resonance imaging (MRI)* has been used increasingly in the abdomen and pelvis, particularly in staging tumours within the pelvis.

## Intravenous urogram (IVU)

### Performing the IVU
The IVU is a relatively simple and non-invasive investigation. A preliminary or control film is initially performed to exclude renal calculi. This is identical to the standard KUB examination and, as such, does not need to be repeated if a KUB has recently been performed. An intravenous injection of a water-soluble iodine-containing contrast medium is then given. Over the subsequent 20–25 minutes a series of films are taken as contrast passes through the kidneys into the ureters and bladder. A compression band is often applied to the mid-abdomen which theoretically compresses the ureters on the adjacent retroperitoneal structures. This helps to distend and maintain the contrast within the upper tracts. Compression is avoided if there has been recent surgery, trauma, or abdominal aortic aneurysm, and in pregnancy. There are few absolute contraindications to performing an IVU, although contrast allergy remains the most important, despite the use of modern contrast media. All radiographic procedures that utilise ionising radiation should be avoided in pregnancy.

### Interpretation of the IVU
Initially, the control films must be evaluated to identify any calcification within the urinary tract. Such calcification would be obscured after injection of contrast medium.

The post-contrast films are then evaluated paying particular attention to the renal position, size and outline, and any distortion of the renal parenchyma. The right kidney usually lies slightly lower than its left-sided counterpart due to its inferior displacement beneath the liver. Renal size is usually measured at between 3 and 4 vertebral bodies in length. The pelvicalyceal system is scrutinised for symmetry, normal filling, and any evidence of extrinsic compression. The ureters are evaluated for size and to ensure free drainage. The bladder is assessed for normal filling and post-micturition emptying.

Careful examination for the presence of any filling defects should be performed.

After reviewing the IVU film series for renal tract pathology, the remainder of the films must be reviewed to exclude alternative pathology. In particular, the bowel gas pattern must be reviewed, and calcified gallstones or aortic aneurysm may be seen. The bones must be examined for degenerative change or metastases. The bases of the lungs are often seen and a lung lesion may very occasionally be identified.

### Intravenous contrast agents

Water-soluble contrast media are widely used in radiology. They are safe but there are a few contraindications to their use, for example *previous allergic reaction* to contrast medium or iodine, *renal failure* and *severe asthma*.

Water-soluble contrast media can very rarely react with metformin, causing lactic acidosis. Thus patients are advised to stop taking metformin for 48 hours after the IVU and have their renal function checked; if these results are normal they can restart metformin.

The major side effects of water-soluble contrast media are anaphylactic hypersensitivity reactions, which can lead to death, cardiovascular compromise due to high osmotic potential of the contrast medium, and contrast-induced nephropathy. All of these are rare. The minor side effects, which occur frequently, are nausea, vomiting, a sensation of warmth, and a metallic taste in the mouth.

## Key points of IVU and urinary tract imaging

- The control films must be reviewed for renal tract calcification (this may be obscured after contrast has been given).
- The kidneys must be examined for position and outline.
- The pelvicalyceal system must be seen to fill normally and ureteric drainage must be confirmed (filling defects may be subtle).
- If the collecting system is obstructed, the site and the degree of obstruction must be assessed.
- A normal IVU takes 25–30 minutes to complete. If films have been taken after this time, it is probably abnormal.
- Other important pathologies may be present on the radiographs.
- The CT KUB has replaced the IVU for the evaluation of renal colic in many centres.
- Ultrasound and CT may be needed for further evaluation of the urinary tract, particularly to diagnose renal obstruction or a renal mass.

## CASE 4.1 Renal tract stones

These three images are KUB (kidneys, ureters, bladder) examinations.

- Image (A) confirms a ureteric calculus at the pyeloureteric junction (arrow).
- Image (B) shows a staghorn calculus (note also a calcified uterine fibroid).
- Image (C) shows bladder calculi (note also calcified gallstone).

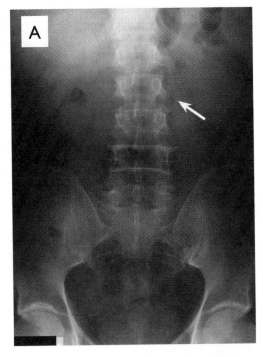

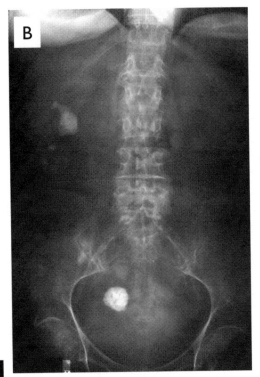

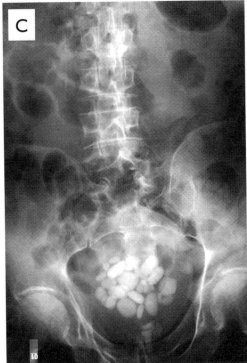

## Background

The KUB will detect 90% of calculi within the urinary tract, and is therefore widely used as a first-line investigation. However, its evaluation can be made difficult if there are large quantities of bowel gas/faeces, calcified costochondral cartilages or calcified arteries, which may obscure small calculi (*Figure 4.1a*). Similarly, calcified phleboliths (calcification within the walls of perivesical veins) can be mistaken for calculi at the vesicoureteric orifices. Phleboliths, however, typically have a 'polo mint' configuration, with a smooth outline, and often a central lucency corresponding to the vein lumen (*Figure 4.1b*).

The importance of the preliminary film cannot be over-emphasised, since small non-obstructing calculi, or even the large staghorn calculi (shown on previous page) may be completely obscured after contrast has been given.

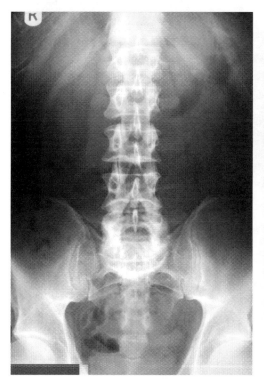 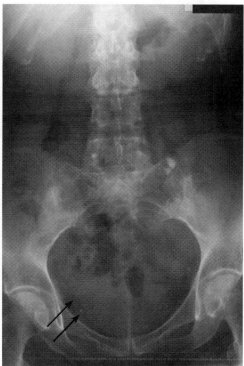

*Figure 4.1a. Calcified costochondral cartilages and faecal loading, which may mimic or obscure small intrarenal or ureteric calculi.*

*Figure 4.1b. Calcified pelvic phleboliths (arrows) overlying the left sacroiliac joint. Note also the presence of calcified costochondral cartilages and lymph nodes.*

## CASE 4.2 Renal tract obstruction due to distal calculus

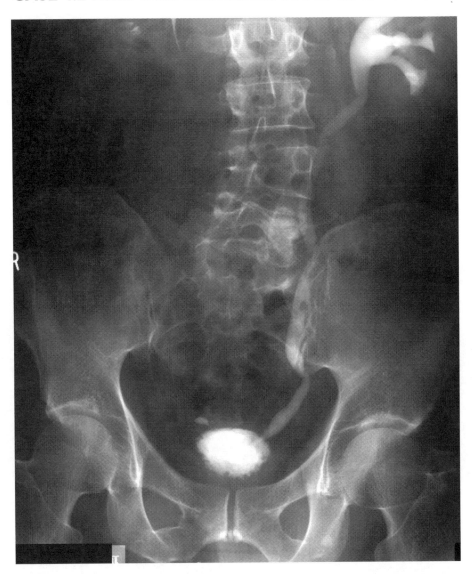

Film from an IVU series demonstrating delayed renal excretion and a standing column of contrast; features due to a calculus at the vesicoureteric orifice, which is now obscured by the excreted contrast.

### Background

The IVU is often performed in cases of suspected renal colic, both to confirm the presence of a calculus, and to assess whether there is obstruction to the renal tract. The importance of the preliminary film cannot be over-emphasised (*Figure 4.2a*) since small non-obstructing calculi may be completely obscured after contrast has been given. The commonest sites of obstruction are at the pelviureteric junction and the vesicoureteric junction.

Partial or complete obstruction of the renal tract results in dilation and a standing column of contrast in the ureter. In complete obstruction, no contrast is seen distal to the obstruction and because of the high pressures created there may be extravasation of contrast from the kidney into the retroperitoneal space (*Figure 4.2b*). Occasionally, the calculus may be passed, but the standing column persists, and only a trickle of contrast is seen to pass into the bladder. This is due to residual oedema at the site of previous stone impaction.

It should be remembered that CT KUB examinations are increasingly being used in place of IVU for stone diagnosis (see *Case 5.13*).

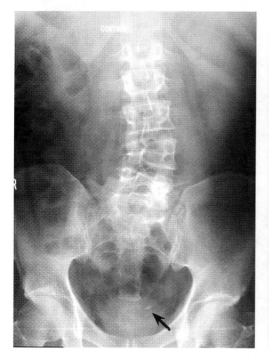

*Figure 4.2a. Control film from the above IVU series showing irregular calcific density at the left vesicoureteric orifice (arrow). Note that this does not appear typical of phlebolith.*

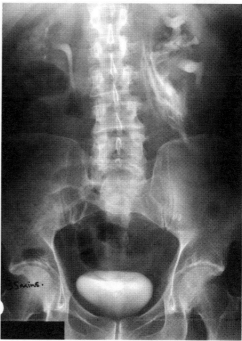

*Figure 4.2b. Film from IVU series demonstrating extravasation of contrast from the kidney into the retroperitoneal space.*

## CASE 4.3 Urinary tract malignancy: renal cell carcinoma

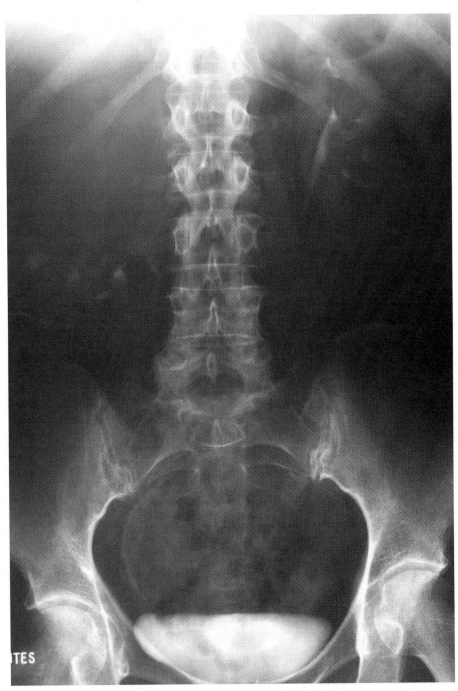

IVU showing distortion and displacement of the pelvicalyceal system in the upper pole of the right kidney, possibly due to a renal mass.

## Background

Malignancy of the kidney or renal tract is a serious cause of macroscopic or microscopic haematuria, and this diagnosis often requires exclusion. A mass within the kidney is manifested on IVU by distortion of the renal outline and/or pelvicalyceal system. This may represent a primary renal cell carcinoma, metastasis (from lung, breast, lymphoma or contralateral kidney), cyst, abscess or benign mass. US is usually performed to exclude a simple cyst as a cause (*Figure 4.3a*), but CT may be needed in further evaluation, and/or staging of a carcinoma (*Figure 4.3b*).

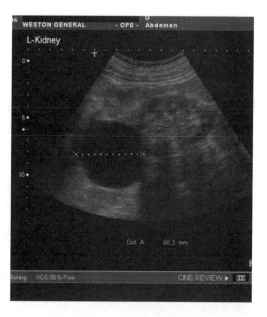

Figure 4.3a. Ultrasound scan of the left kidney demonstrating a large simple renal cyst.

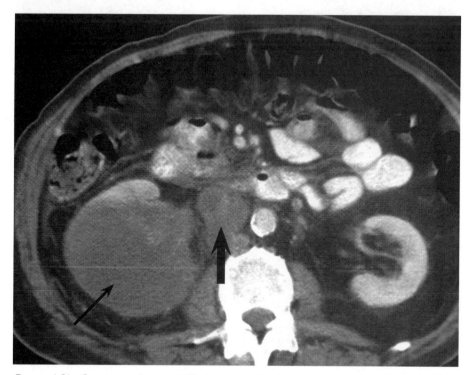

Figure 4.3b. Contrast-enhanced CT showing mixed-density mass due to renal cell carcinoma involving the entirety of the right kidney (thin arrow). There is involvement of the IVC and adjacent lymph nodes (thick arrow).

## CASE 4.4 Urinary tract malignancy: transitional cell carcinoma

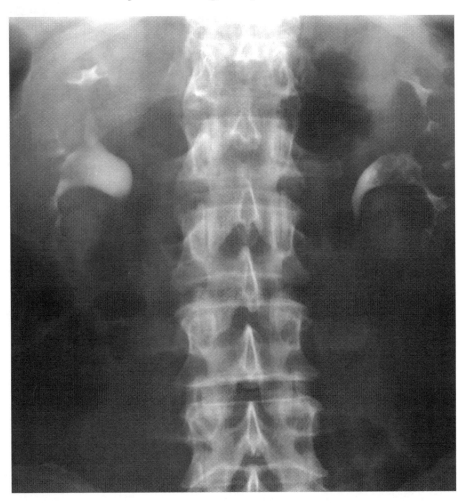

IVU showing irregular filling defects within the left pelvicalyceal system due to transitional cell carcinoma.

## Background

TCCs may occur at any site of urothelial epithelium, within the renal collecting system (as in *Case 4.4*) or within the bladder or ureter. These tumours are seen on IVU as irregular filling defects within these structures. Depending on the size and position of the TCC they may obstruct the renal tract, causing hydronephrosis (*Figure 4.4a*) or hydroureter (*Figure 4.4b*).

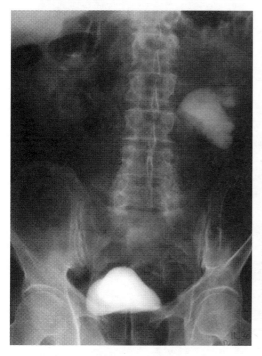

*Figure 4.4a. IVU showing large irregular filling defect within the renal pelvis causing hydronephrosis.*

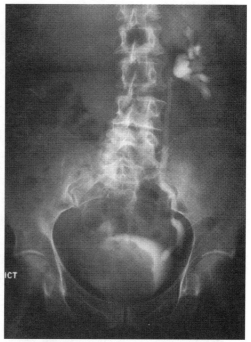

*Figure 4.4b. IVU showing irregular filling defects within the right side of the bladder, in keeping with TCC. There is complete loss in function on this side with no contrast excretion from the right kidney. Note the left-sided hydroureter and hydronephrosis. These are caused by the bladder mass which must also be impinging upon the left vesicoureteric orifice.*

## CASE 4.5 Rare filling defects

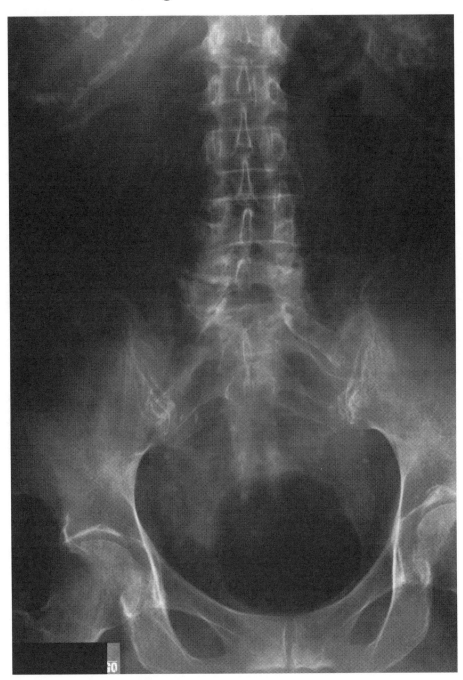

KUB examination showing gas density (black) within the bladder and pelv-calyceal systems. There is a differential diagnosis for these appearances as discussed on the following page.

## Background

Gas in the urinary tract is an uncommon but important diagnosis. Gas bubbles are seen as filling defects in the urinary tract on the IVU examination. These small lucencies may be visible on the control film and may be differentiated from bowel gas by their position and shape within the collecting system.

The differential diagnosis for such gas includes:

- *Infections*: gas-forming organisms such as *Escherichia coli*.
- *Fistulae*: due to diverticular disease, carcinoma of the bowel or Crohn's disease.
- *Iatrogenic (urinary diversion, instrumentation) and penetrating wounds*: if this has occurred due to infection, gas may also be seen in the renal parenchyma (emphysematous pyelonephritis) extending into the retroperitoneal tissues.

There may also be gas in the bladder wall (emphysematous cystitis – not seen here).

Renal calculi and TCC are the two commonest causes of filling defects in the urinary tract. Other causes include:

- Other malignancies (squamous cell carcinoma, metastases), blood clot.
- Sloughed papilla (eg. due to diabetes mellitus, or due to non-steroidal analgesics).
- Fungus balls.
- Gas bubbles (as seen here).

## CASE 4.6 Congenital abnormalities of the renal tract

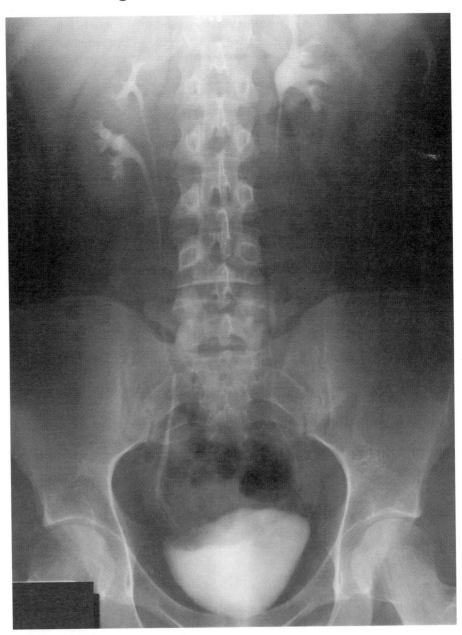

IVU showing a duplex collecting system and ureter.

## Background

*Complete or incomplete duplication* of a ureter is not uncommon. 1 in 500 of the population have complete ureteric duplication, the incidence of incomplete duplication being higher. Duplication of the ureter is often an incidental finding on an IVU, but they can be complicated by vesicoureteric reflux or recurrent infections.

A *ureterocele* is a submucosal dilation of the intravesical ureter. Ureterocele occurs in the asymtomatic population at a frequency of 1 in 5000 to 1 in 12 000. They are often associated with a duplex ureteric system. On IVU this is seen as a smooth-walled contrast-filled structure surrounded by a radiolucent rim, which itself is surrounded by contrast in the bladder. This has been called the 'cobra's head' sign (*Figure 4.6a*). Ureteroceles are often asymptomatic incidental findings but they can be associated with calculi, infections or obstruction.

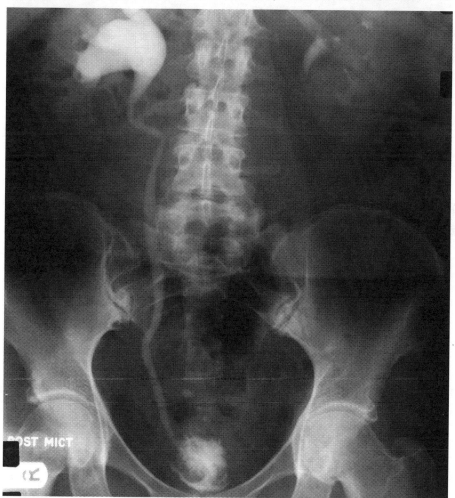

## CASE 4.7 Extrinsic mass lesions

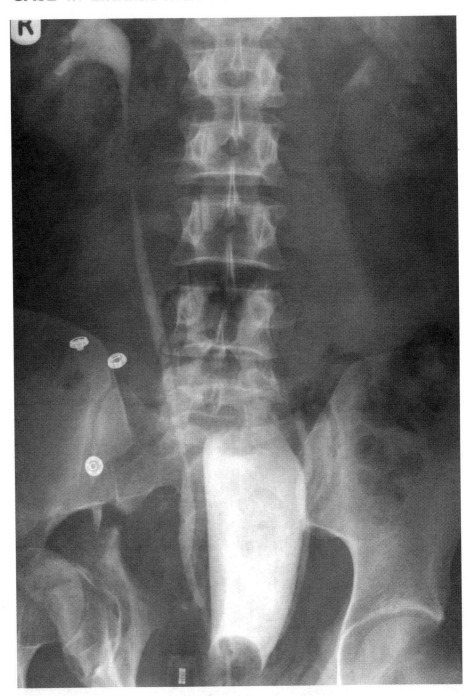

IVU showing distortion of the bladder due to pelvic haematoma – in this case due to a displaced right acetabular fracture.

## Background

The IVU sometimes provides information on pathologies outside the renal tract. A mass outside the renal tract may distort it from its normal position. A pelvic mass, for example, can distort the normal shape of the bladder.

Similar appearances may occur due to any of the following:

- abscess
- ovarian mass
- enlarged prostate
- hepatomegaly causing renal displacement and distortion.

## CASE 4.8 Horseshoe kidney

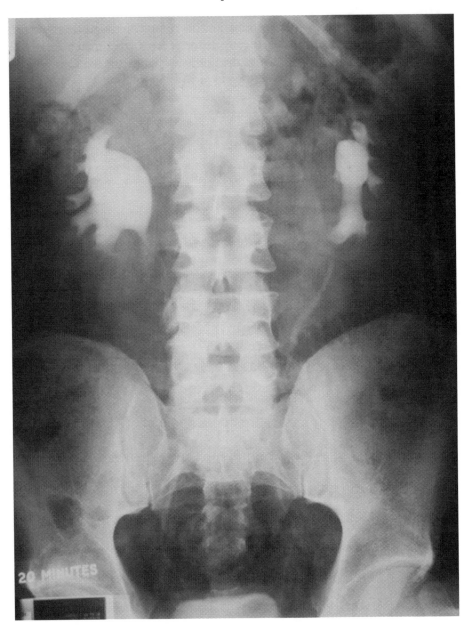

This film taken at 20 minutes from an IVU series demonstrates that both kidneys are abnormally orientated with medial deviation of their lower poles. There is also mild bilateral hydronephrosis. These are the appearances of a horseshoe kidney.

## Background

Horseshoe kidney is a congenital abnormality whereby the lower poles of both kidneys remain fused to one another, either by a fibrous link, or due to renal tissue. It is well demonstrated on CT (*Figure 4.8a*). As a result, the kidneys lie in an abnormal orientation, and are more prone to trauma. Furthermore, horseshoe kidneys are susceptible to outflow obstruction since the ureters originate anteriorly from the renal collecting system and then pass anterior to the inferior part of the horseshoe.

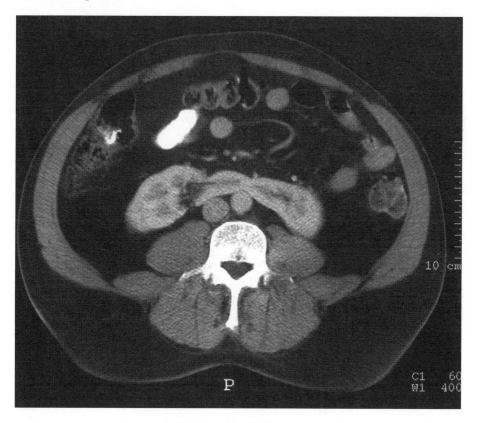

*Figure 4.8a. CT scan confirming horseshoe kidney, with enhancing renal parenchyma uniting the lower poles of both kidneys.*

# Section 5

## I: Ultrasound
## II: Computed Tomography
## III: Magnetic Resonance Imaging

## PART I ULTRASOUND

## Introduction

It would be extremely unusual to be presented with an ultrasound scan in a medical finals examination, but should that happen this section will be invaluable. The aim of this section is primarily to enable the reader confronted with an ultrasound examination to recognise it as such, and to be able to discuss the basics of ultrasound (US), including its main uses and limitations.

### How to recognise a US scan

Your first impression of a US scan may be that it is totally unrecognisable, and although some people may rely on this fact ('Well it certainly isn't MR or CT and it all looks rather blurred, so I think it must be ultrasound') we will give a reasonably foolproof method of approach.

US probes are usually (for the purposes of this text, but unfortunately not always) curved on the edge which is placed against the patient's body surface. As a result, the image will usually have a curved upper edge. There is also a fan-like configuration of the image due to divergance of the US beam. These are certain indicators of US (*Figure 5-I.A*).

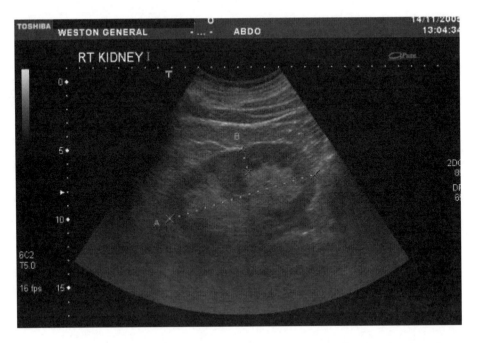

*Figure 5-I.A. US of right kidney. Note the curved upper edge and fan-shaped configuration of the image. Note also that the organ has been annotated and measured.*

### The basics of ultrasound scanning

US depends upon echoes generated from the probe passing into the body and then being bounced back (reflected) or absorbed within the tissues. The pattern of echoes that arrives back at the transducer is then computer-processed to form an image. The US waves do not pass through air, and so ultrasound gel is required to couple the transducer to the skin surface. Accordingly, US cannot be used to evaluate any air-containing viscus (eg. bowel or lung) due to the gas within these structures. Likewise, US waves do not pass through bone. Due to these limitations, US is primarily used to evaluate the soft tissue viscera of the upper abdomen, blood vessels (eg. aorta or peripheral venous structures for thrombus), chest if pleural fluid is present, or more superficial soft tissue structures (eg. testis, thyroid) and superficial musculoskeletal structures.

The overwhelming advantage of US is that it does not rely upon radiation, but its disadvantages include operator variability, the body habitus of the patient, and the fact that excessively gas-filled bowel may obscure the underlying soft tissue structures. In addition, the US examination is a dynamic study; with the operator continuously evaluating the scan during the 5 to 10 minutes required to perform it. As a result, the single images obtained from the examination are only snapshots from the overall study and a review of them in the absence of the operator may be misleading (just as half a dozen photographs may not be a true representation of a short film).

### Nomenclature in ultrasound scanning

In CT different gradations of grey are described as low or high density; in US these are referred to as areas of low or high echogenicity – black or white, respectively.

An echogenic structure such as a gallstone will create a shadow behind it, since the nature of the stone will prevent US waves from passing through it (*Figure 5-I.B*). This is known as an acoustic shadow, and tends to be seen in dense structures such as bone or calculi (including gallstones).

Similarly, an area of fluid density is usually of low echogenicity, and allows a greater proportion of US waves to pass through it. As a result the tissues behind such a structure will be exposed to a less attenuated beam. This is known as acoustic enhancement, and it is characteristic of a cyst to give this appearance.

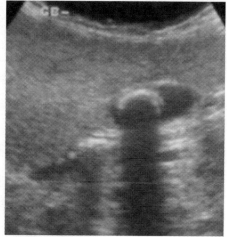

*Figure 5-I.B. US of single gallstone within gallbladder, with associated acoustic shadow.*

It should therefore be apparent that dense structures such as calculi tend to be echogenic (white) and fluid tends to be of low echogenicity (dark). Fat also tends to be quite attenuating to the US beam, although not as much as a calcified structure, and fat will not usually cause acoustic shadowing to the same extent. Normal soft tissues are of mixed echogenicity (various shades of intermediate grey).

A Doppler US (also referred to as 'colour Doppler') refers to a particular function of the US machine that detects movement. This modality of US is primarily used for vascular examinations. Flow is depicted as either red or blue on the image, depending on whether the movement is towards or away from the transducer. The colour (red or blue) does not depend upon the velocity, or whether the structure is arterial or venous, but purely on the direction with respect to the probe. Hence an artery or vein may appear red or blue depending upon the position of the probe (*Figure 5-I.Ca and b*). A duplex US is a variant of the above, whereby the vessel is depicted in two formats on the screen. Half of the screen shows colour flow, as described above, but the operator also places a cursor at a particular position within the vessel to sample and depict the velocity waveform in graph format.

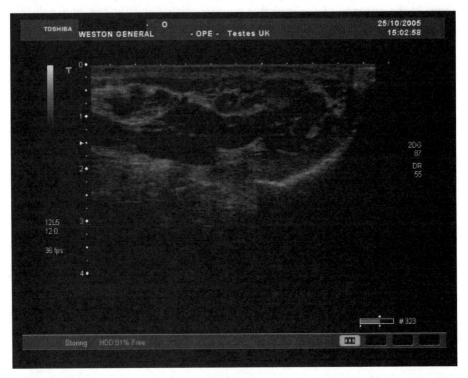

*Figure 5-I.Ca. US of left testicular varicocele showing low echogenicity within the distended venous plexus.*

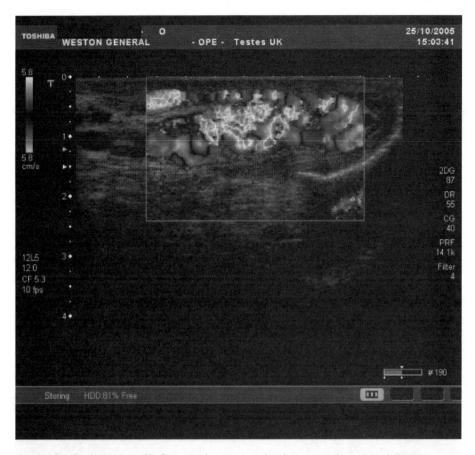

*Figure 5-I.Cb. Doppler of left testicular varicocele showing colour signal due to venous flow.*

Instead of the case format presented elsewhere in this book, this section will now demonstrate a series of examples of classical ultrasound diagnoses (*Cases 5.1–5.9*).

| Key points of ultrasound |
|---|
| Understand the following terms: |
| ■ High or low echogenicity.<br>■ Acoustic shadow.<br>■ Acoustic enhancement.<br>■ Doppler and duplex. |

## CASE 5.1 Acute cholecystitis

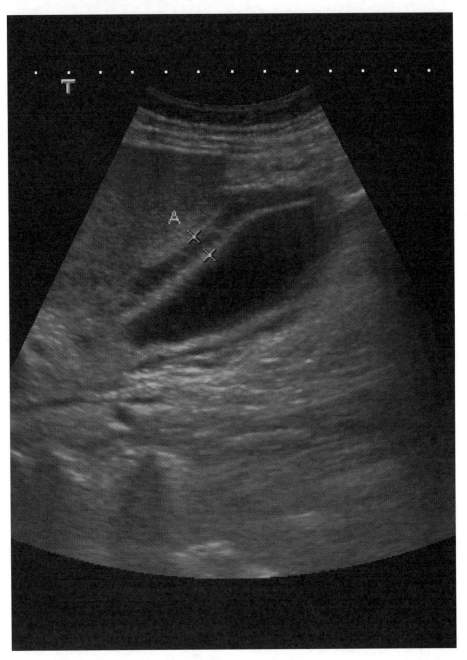

There is marked thickening of the gallbladder wall. Stones are usually also seen (not seen on this actual image) and localised tenderness over the gallbladder (the so-called ultrasound McMurphy sign) is also often elicited at the time of the scan.

## CASE 5.2 Hydronephrosis

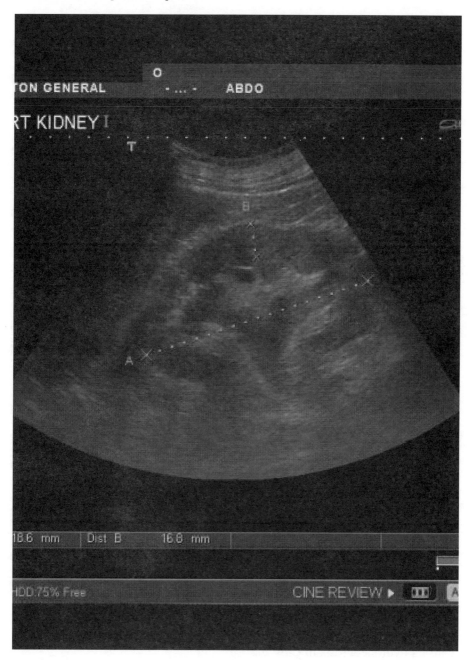

Note the distension of the renal collecting system, appearing as low echogenicity fluid.

## CASE 5.3 Fluid-filled cyst

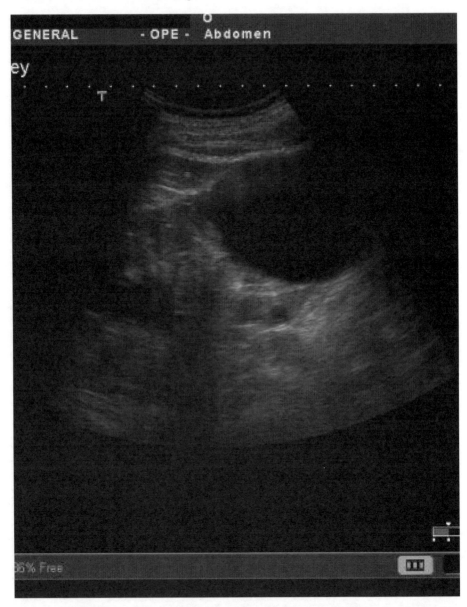

US showing a fluid-filled cyst (seen as the same echogenicity as the urine causing hydronephrosis in *Case 5.2)*.

## CASE 5.4 Renal cell carcinoma

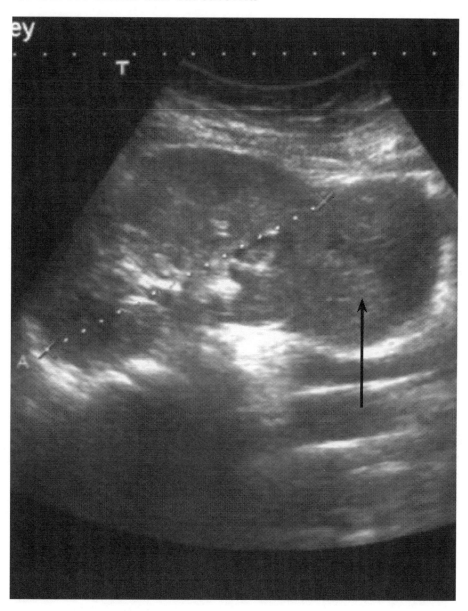

US showing a mixed-echogenicity mass arising within the kidney (arrow). This is most likely to represent a renal cell carcinoma.

## CASE 5.5 Abdominal aortic aneurysm

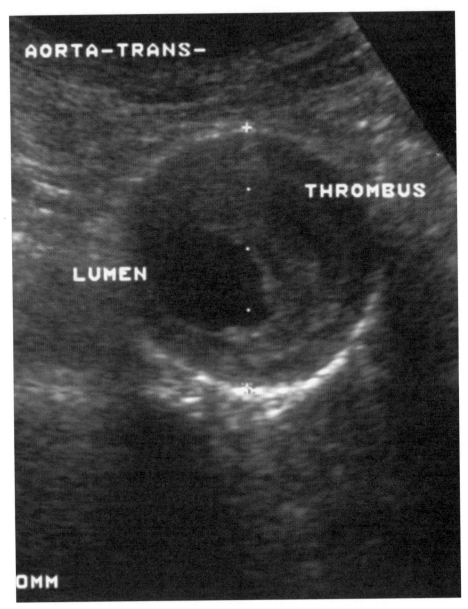

US demonstrating a transverse section through an abdominal aortic aneurysm. Note the presence of intramural thrombus.

## CASE 5.6 Ascites

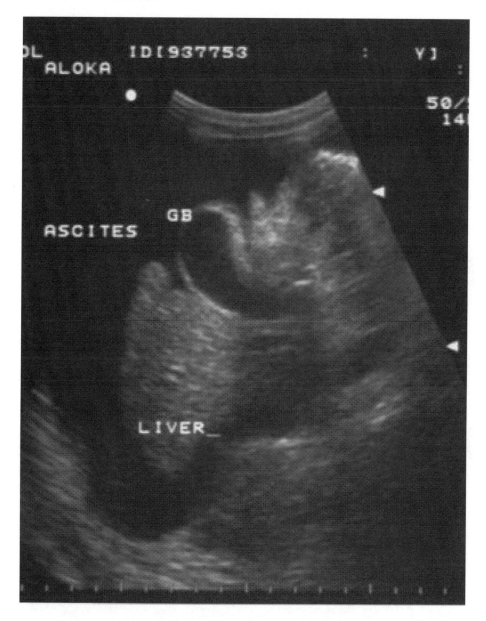

US confirming the presence of ascites. As in the previous cases, fluid is seen as low echogenicity. Note the liver and other tissues annotated on the image. Pleural fluid would give similar appearances within the chest.

## CASE 5.7 Ultrasound of the testis

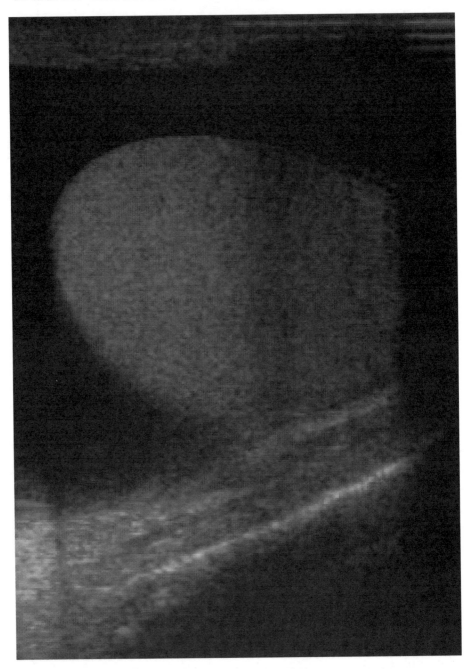

Ultrasound is particularly useful for the evaluation of the testes since these structures are both superficial and radiation sensitive. This image is an US of the testis showing normal testicular echogenicity. There is a large amount of surrounding fluid (black area) due to the presence of a hydrocoele.

## CASE 5.8 Deep venous thrombosis

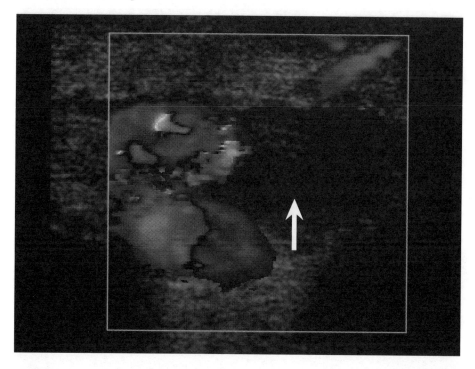

US of the iliofemoral vein at the groin, performed with colour Doppler. Note the lack of vein compressibility and the lack of colour flow in keeping with extensive thrombus (arrow). The mixed echogenicity seen adjacent to this is due to colour flow within the femoral artery.

## CASE 5.9 Ultrasound of the pelvis

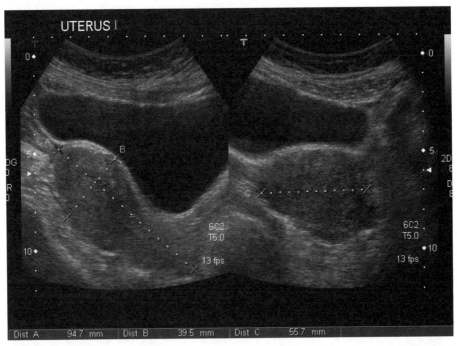

Ultrasound of the pelvis showing urine within the bladder and normal uterus. Ultrasound is commonly used in evaluation of the pelvis where ionising radiation should be avoided if possible due to the sensitivity of the pelvic organs to radiation.

# PART II COMPUTED TOMOGRAPHY

## Introduction

The aim of this section is primarily to enable readers confronted with a CT scan in an examination situation to begin their description as impressively as possible (This is a CT scan of the abdomen of John Smith, aged 50. It has been performed with both intravenous and oral contrast. I will now review the normal anatomy as follows…') Examples of some pathology are given in this section, but it is beyond the limitations and needs of this book to review anything more than easily interpretable abnormalities. *Cases 5.10–5.16* show some classical computed tomograpy (CT) diagnoses.

### The principles of CT

CT scanning involves a bank of X-ray-producing tubes with a corresponding array of detectors on the far side of the patient. The tubes and detectors rotate around the patient as the tubes emit an X-ray beam composed of several hundred radiation pulses. The X-rays pass through the patient and are then detected. The computed analysis of the information derived from each of the detectors in turn results in the formation of axial images (cross-sectional slices) of the anatomical site of interest. This can be likened to a light giving a series of shadows of any three-dimensional structure. The analysis of these shadows will ultimately allow an image of that structure to be made. The larger the number of shadows available for analysis, the more detailed the final image will be.

The original, simple *axial scanners* performed a series of scans at one level, which would allow the formation of a single axial image. The scanner would then move the patient further into the scanner and repeat the scan at the next level. More recent scanners perform a *spiral* of scans as the patient moves through them in a continuous nature. This development in scan technique occurred due to the arrival of slip-ring technology. The most recent generation of scanners work in a similar way, but a series of detectors (usually 4 or 16, but sometimes now 32 or even 64) are used to allow greater detail and speed. These are called *multislice scanners*.

### How to recognise a CT scan

Students often ask how to differentiate between a CT and an MR scan. Unfortunately, due to the variety of different signal intensities that may be generated on MR, this may be a difficult differentiation to make for the non-radiologist. A reliable means of discrimination is, however, described below.

CT scanning depends upon radiation pulses, followed by computer processing to form an image. The radiation pulses originate from an X-ray tube within the scanner. X-rays are produced in the X-ray tube with a particular voltage and current. This is not the case in magnetic resonance imaging (MRI). A CT scan will always have these values annotated on each scan as Kv and mAS. (See *Figure 5-II.A*). Conversely, MRI may be recognised by annotations such as TE, TR, FLAIR, and STIR (see *Section 5-III*).

### Multiplanar reconstructions (MPRs) and more sophisticated image manipulation

The improved image resolution and speed of image acquisition possible with modern multislice CT scanners allows narrower and more detailed images to be obtained. As a result, a series of axial images can be computer analysed to be viewed as coronal, sagittal or oblique reconstructions in addition to the standard axial orientation. This is known as multiplanar reconstruction (MPR).

Furthermore, parts of a scan may be 'cut away' to allow clearer imaging of the region of interest. For example, the images of renal artery stenosis (see *Figure 5-II.A*) were obtained by performing an initial narrow section axial image through the renal arteries during an arterial phase of contrast injection. This volume acquisition was manipulated coronally, and then further image rendering performed to allow specific analysis of the renal arteries.

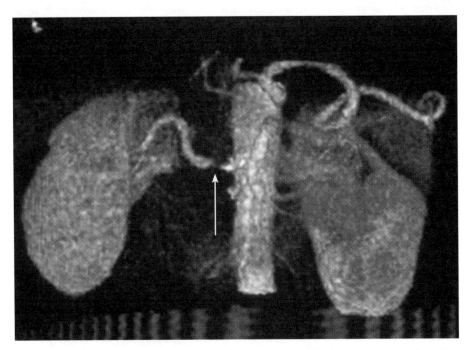

Figure 5-II.A. Multiplanar reconstruction in coronal plane accentuating the appearance of a right renal artery stenosis (arrow).

### Interpretation of the CT scan

This section covers the basic principles of scan interpretation, and includes the orientation of the patient within the scanner, whether or not contrast has been given, and some basic anatomy. The Key Points list for this section (p. 183) provides some 'good words to use' in the description of a CT scan, which if used appropriately may impress your examiners! Some examples of pathology will then be discussed.

### Patient orientation in CT scanning

For standard scanning of the chest, abdomen pelvis or brain, the scans are invariably printed as if the viewer were at the foot of the patient's bed, looking up through the patient in sequential slices. Thus, the scan is seen as shown in (*Figure 5-II.B*).

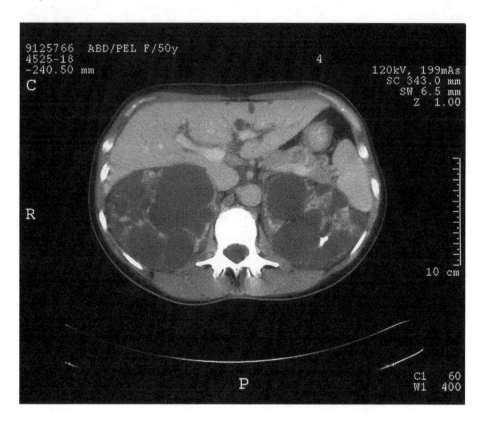

*Figure 5-II.B. CT of the abdomen with right (R) and posterior (P) markers on each scan slice. Note therefore the position of the vertebral bodies and spinous processes posteriorly. Kv and mAS are also annotated on the scan, confirming this is a CT image. This scan shows incidental polycystic kidney disease.*

### Contrast in CT

Contrast may be either oral or intravenous in its route of administration. The exact nature of the contrast to be used will be decided by the radiologist according to the clinical information on the request.

*Oral contrast* is usually either barium sulphate or an iodine-containing compound (eg. Gastromiro® or Gastrografin®). The presence (or not) of oral contrast can be determined by reviewing the loops of bowel on the abdominal scan, where contrast is seen as areas of high density (white) (see *Figure 5-II.C*).

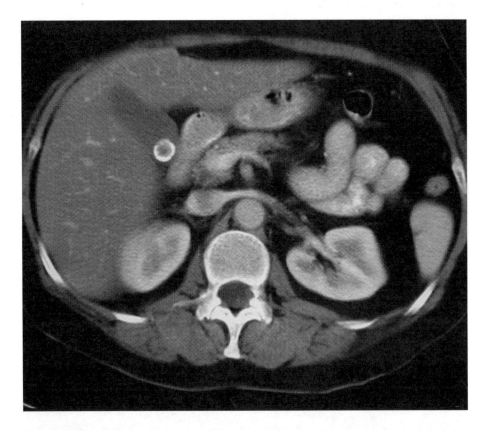

*Figure 5-II.C. CT of the abdomen after oral contrast has been administered, showing contrast within the loops of small and large bowel. Note the incidental presence of a calcified gallstone within the gallbladder.*

*Intravenous contrast* is given by injection through a venous cannula normally in the antecubital fossa. The contrast passes into the right side of the heart, through the lungs and then to the left ventricle and aorta. The timing of this passage is variable according to the patient's individual cardiac output, but is usually in the region of 15 seconds for reaching the pulmonary artery, and 20 seconds for the aorta. From then, the contrast returns either through the inferior vena cava or via the portal vein to the liver (approximately 45–60 seconds post initial injection). The scan is therefore timed according to the structures that require maximum opacification. For example, a CT pulmonary angiogram will be performed between 10 and 20 seconds after the commencement of the injection, when there is maximum contrast opacification to the pulmonary artery and its branches.

The contrast itself is usually injected using a mechanised pump, in order to deliver suitable volume in the time allowed time (eg. 100 mL in 25 seconds) and to avoid the need for the operator to be in the scanner itself (thus avoiding radiation exposure).

The presence (or not) of intravenous contrast is easiest to determine by reviewing the aorta or IVC, where contrast is seen to fill the lumen as a region of high density (white) (see *Figure 5-II.D*).

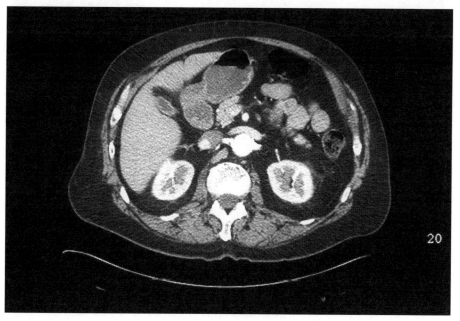

*Figure 5-II.D. CT of the abdomen after intravenous contrast has been injected, showing contrast enhancement within the lumen of the aorta.*

In the evaluation of a CT of the brain, the presence of contrast is detected by the presence of opacification within the vessels of the circle of Willis (*Figure 5-II.E*). Perhaps more simply, the majority of radiology departments will also put a small '+c' (ie. plus contrast) within the other nomenclature on each axial slice of an IV contrast-enhanced CT.

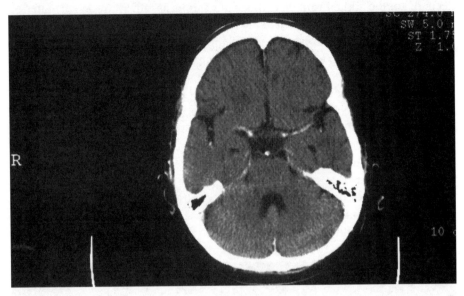

Figure 5-I.E. CT of the brain after intravenous contrast has been injected, showing contrast enhancement within the circle of Willis.

### Centering and windowing values in CT

Any CT scan is depicted as a cross-sectional slice. This is portrayed as a grey series (ie. from black to white with an intermediate grey range). The degree of greyness is determined by the density of the structure. This concept was first developed by Hounsfield, and therefore each pixel on the scan can be given a density value (known as the Hounsfield unit, HU, for that area). The HU figures range between –1000 and +1000, with water being 1, and air and bone being between –500 to –1000 and +500 to +1000, respectively.

Within the body, there is too great a variety of tissue densities (eg. between bone and lung) for all structures to be meaningfully depicted on a single grey scale; in other words if a single grey scale were used to encompass –1000 (air in lung) to +1000 (bone in lumbar spine) then there would be insufficient intermediate shades of grey to determine such a huge density range, and subtle changes in tissue density would not be visible. Therefore, any scan can be viewed according to the setting of windows (centred at a particular level with a range on either side) to concentrate on the densities of interest within the region scanned. In reality these are often preset on the scanner.

Therefore, if, the chest is scanned, for example, the images can be evaluated on a lung window (to evaluate the lungs), then on an abdominal window (to evaluate the soft tissues of the mediastinum) and a bone window (to review the vertebral bodies and ribs). This can all be done after the single scan has been performed, in post-scan processing (*Figures 5-II.F to 5-II.H*).

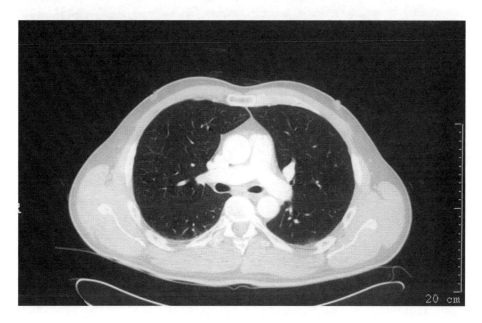

*Figure 5-II.F. CT of the chest, viewed on chest window.*

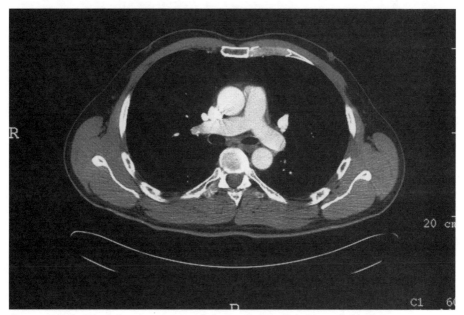

*Figure 5-II.G. CT of the chest, viewed on mediastinal/abdominal window.*

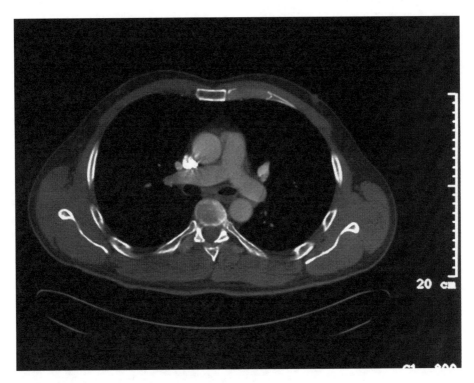

Figure 5-II.H. CT of the chest, viewed on bone window.

## CT scan of normal anatomy

The abdominal viscera can be seen on the annotated CT scan in *Figure 5-II.I.*

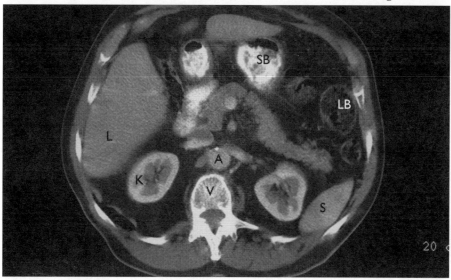

*Figure 5-II.I. Normal anatomy of the abdominal viscera. The kidneys (K) lie on either side of the midline in the retroperitoneal areas. They normally enhance well on the injection of intravenous contrast. The liver (L) and spleen (S) have similar densities within the upper abdomen. The liver is supplied in greater part by the portal vein, and therefore scanning of this organ is best performed at 60 seconds after intravenous contrast injection if metastases are being sought. The aorta (A) lies in a retroperitoneal position, just to the left of the midline, an terior to the vertebral bodies (V). The aorta scanned in arterial phase will appear of high density due to the intravenous contrast within it. The appearances of the small (SB) and large bowel (LB) are variable according to how much oral contrast they contain, the amount of faecal loading or fluid distention within the bowel, and the time of scanning after the oral contrast was administered. If the entirety of small and large bowel is required to be opacified (as is often the case for abdomen and pelvis scans) then bowel contrast should be given 1–2 hours before the scan takes place. If this is not done, then unopacified loops of bowel may be difficult to differentiate, and small collections of blood, pus or fluid may not be appreciated. Similarly, bowel-related masses (eg. colonic tumours) may not be seen.*

---

### Key points of computed tomography

These are also 'good words to use' when describing a CT scan.
- Density: low (black/dark grey), intermediate or high (white/light grey).
- Contrast: oral or intravenous.
- Phase of the scan: arterial (pulmonary or aortic) or portal venous (look for contrast within the liver).
- Windowing levels.
- Abnormal mass arising within (for example) the kidney…on the left side (saying this shows you know about the orientation of the scan).

## CASE 5.10 Abdominal aortic aneurysm

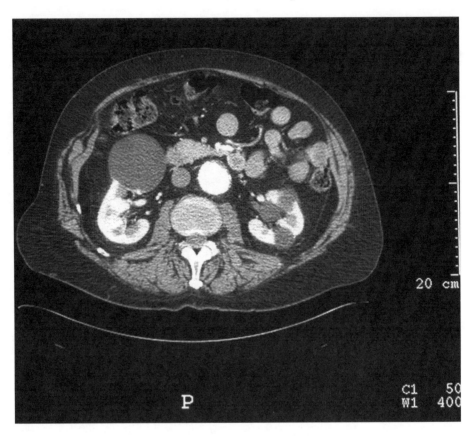

20 cm

C1   50
W1   400

P

CT scan of the abdomen, performed with oral and intravenous contrast, demonstrating the presence of an abdominal aortic aneurysm. Note the presence of a small amount of thrombus within the lumen on the anterior wall and multiple incidental renal cysts. The size of the aneurysm may be judged by counting the gradations on the right side of the scan to be approximately 3.5 cm in an antero-posterior dimension. Accurate measurement may be performed on the CT console with measurement cursors.

## CASE 5.11 Small bowel obstruction

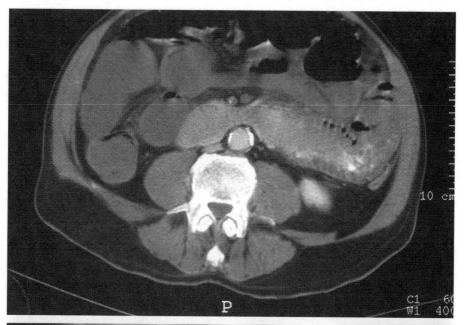

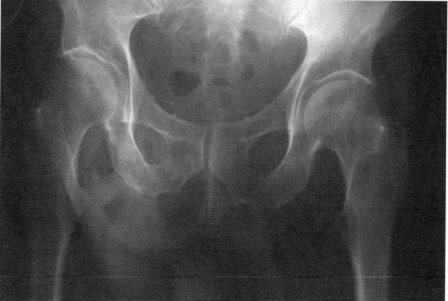

CT scan of the abdomen, performed with oral and intravenous contrast, demonstrating the presence of small bowel obstruction. Note the mild dilation of the small bowel which contains a mixture of contrast and fluid. The cause for these appearances is seen on the lower image as an inguinal hernia. (See also *Case 2.11*).

## CASE 5.12 Pulmonary embolism

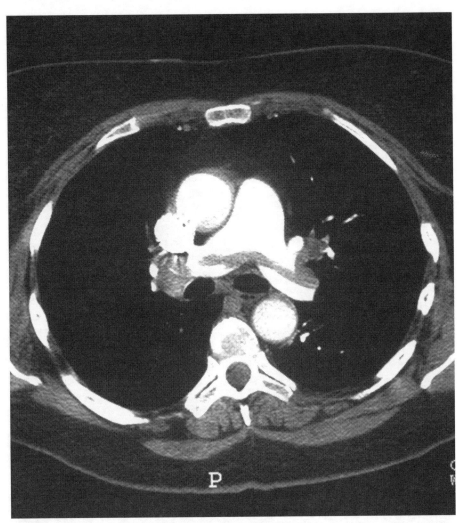

CT pulmonary angiogram (CTPA) performed with intravenously injected contrast and scanned in pulmonary artery phase. This scan demonstrates the presence of a large saddle embolus, which is seen as a large filling defect within the pulmonary trunk, bridging across the origins of the left and right pulmonary arteries. For a full discussion on the evaluation of potential pulmonary embolism see *Case 1.17.*

## CASE 5.13 Renal tract calculi

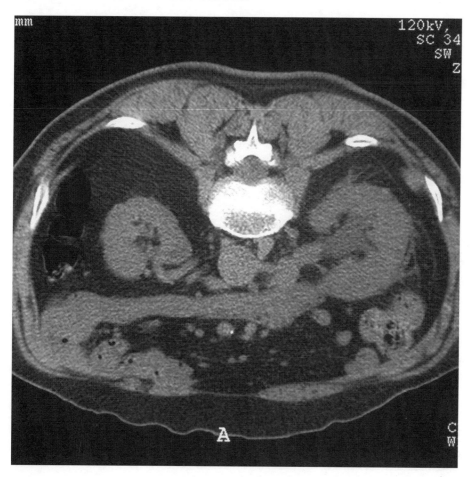

CT scan of the abdomen, but actually localised to the region of the urinary tract. This is a CT KUB (kidneys, ureter and bladder). The examination is performed without intravenous or oral contrast, in order to diagnose the presence of renal tract stones. The right kidney is enlarged and there is adjacent linear stranding with evidence of hydronephrosis. Further discussion of renal tract calculi can be found in *Case 4.2*.

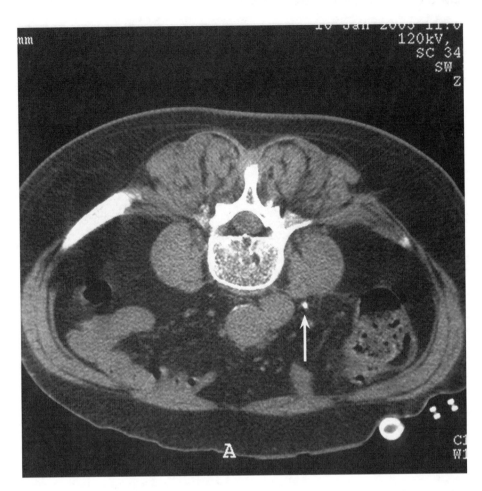

This scan demonstrates the presence of a radiodense ureteric calculus (arrow) lying at the lower limit of the dilated ureter. Note this is an exception to the rule of patients lying supine for the scan to be performed; this scan is perfomed prone so that a stone that has passed into the bladder will fall anteriorly away from the region of the vesicoureteric junction.

## CASE 5.14 Renal cell carcinoma

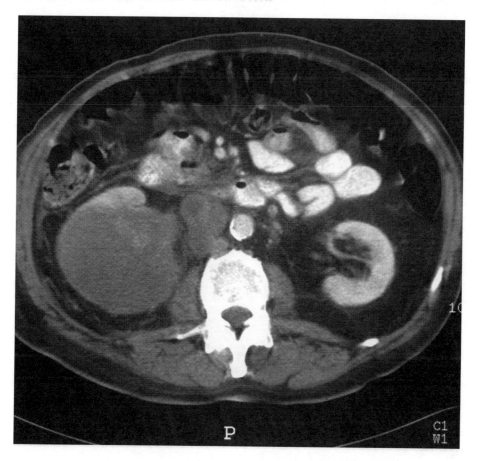

CT scan of the abdomen, performed with oral and intravenous contrast, demonstrating the presence of a large right renal mass with extension into the inferior vena cava (IVC) and adjacent lymphadenopathy.

## CASE 5.15 Lung carcinoma

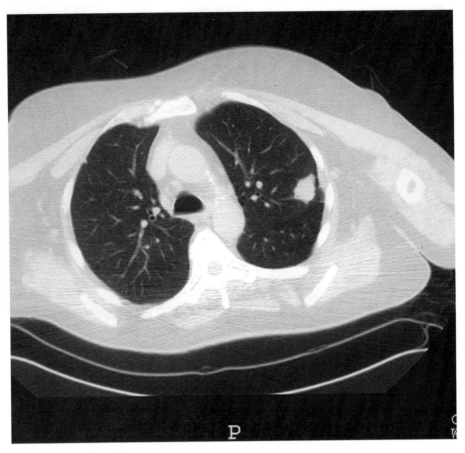

CT scan of the thorax, viewed here on lung window settings. There is a spiculated soft-tissue mass in keeping with primary bronchogenic carcinoma.

## CASE 5.16 Lung metastases

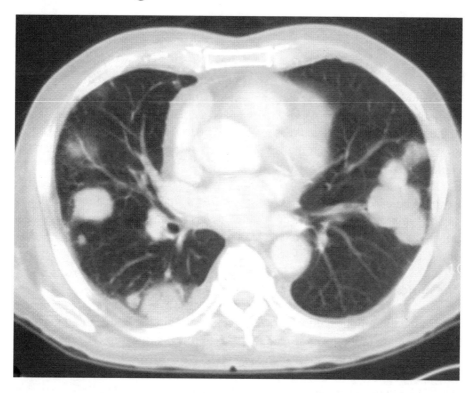

CT scan of the chest demonstrating the presence of multiple abnormal soft tissue densities in keeping with lung metastases.

## PART III MAGNETIC RESONANCE IMAGING (MRI)

## Introduction

MRI imaging is now widely used across most body systems, but in particular in the evaluation of the central nervous and musculoskeletal systems, and now increasingly for performing staging examinations of the pelvis in cases of prostatic, rectal or other pelvic malignancy. In addition, magnetic resonance in the form of cholangiopancreatography (MRCP) and angiography (MRA) is now often used to replace the invasive procedures of endoscopic retrograde cholangiopancreatography (ERCP) and peripheral angiography.

It is beyond the scope of this book to fully discuss the details of MR imaging. It would be exceptionally unlikely for a medical finals examination to include any MR images. However, we do briefly discuss the background of the physical principles involved, how to recognise an MR image, and the advantages and disadvantages of this modality. Several case examples are then presented.

### The basics of MR physics

Due to the ubiquitous nature of hydrogen ions within the body, and their high charge to mass ratio, the hydrogen ion is used for MR imaging. The nucleus of the hydrogen atom contains a single proton. Protons are positively charged and constantly spinning on their axes and therefore induce a surrounding magnetic field. When hydrogen ions are placed in a magnetic field and radiofrequencies are applied, then different tissue types respond differently. It is the detection and measurement of these different responses from the different tissues which allows the construction of an MR image.

If a magnetic force is applied to the body, protons align themselves within the magnetic field. However, they do this by spinning around the axis of the field (precessing) and also by aligning themselves into either a high or low energy state.

A radiofrequency pulse of the same frequency as the precessing protons is then applied and this transfers energy to these protons. This radiofrequency pulse raises the energy levels within the hydrogen ions, and also causes them to precess *in phase*. When the radiofrequency pulse is turned off, the hydrogen ions flip back to a low energy state and slowly come out of phase, and as they do so energy is released in the form of two parts: T1 which represents flipping of hydrogen protons back to a low energy state, and T2 as they come out of phase. Water and fluids tend to have long T1 and T2 times, while fat and more complex molecules have shorter T1 and T2 times. The differences in T1 are largely due to differences in tissue composition and structure, which are also important in determining T2 times where the external magnetic field inhomogeneity is also important.

The magnetic signals produced by the above processes are very small. In addition, the radiofrequency signals produced may at least in part be in the same overall alignment as the magnetic field by the magnet itself, and therefore are impossible to detect. In order to accentuate the small signals and to render them detectable, the radiofrequency is repeated after long or short times, and different strengths of radiofrequency are used. By combination of these techniques the so-called T1-and T2- weighted images are formed.

*A T1-weighted image results in fat as intermediate or high signal (white), and a T2-weighted image results in fluid (hence CSF and urine) as a high signal.*

The overall position of the particular area of tissues sampled is determined by gradients in the overall magnetic field, and by different parts of the body being put in phase or out of phase. Slice thickness can be determined by the gradiant in the external magnetic field.

Magnetic resonance contrast may also be used (gadolinium). This may be used in magnetic resonance arteriography or venography, although sequences have also been developed which allow blood flow to be imaged without the use of any contrast material. These are known as the 'time of flight' sequences. Fast sequences of MR imaging have also been performed. These usually involve use of different types of radiofrequency.

### How to recognise an MR image

The failsafe method is to look for the physical parameters of the scan (in a similar way to CT scan recognition). The variables here are the time to echo (TE) and the time to repeat of echo (TR). Other clues may be from specific image sequences (eg. FLAIR and STIR), which may also be annotated on the scan (*Figure 5-III.A*). (Remember that these anotations will not always appear on individual images)

---

**Key points of magnetic resonance imaging**

Note the advantages of MRI:

- Avoids use of ionising radiation.
- Excellent soft-tissue evaluation (therefore used in musculoskeletal imaging).
- Good fluid evaluation with MRCP and MRA (Figures 5-III.B and 5-III.C).
- Capacity for 3-D manipulation and representation (therefore used to show sagittal images of the spine as in Figure 5-III.D).
- Remember also the disadvantages: patients cannot be scanned if they have cardiac implants such as pacemakers or defibrillators since the magnetic field may cause them to malfunction. Similarly, metallic foreign bodies (eg. intra-orbital) should be excluded.
- Time-consuming scanning techniques (but reduced by time-saving protocols).
- Specialist supportive equipment is needed for unstable patients (strong magnetic fields preclude use of standard anaesthetic equipment in ventilated patients).
- May cause distress to patients with claustrophobia (because of the proximity of the scanner surrounding the patient and the noise it produces).

## MR brain

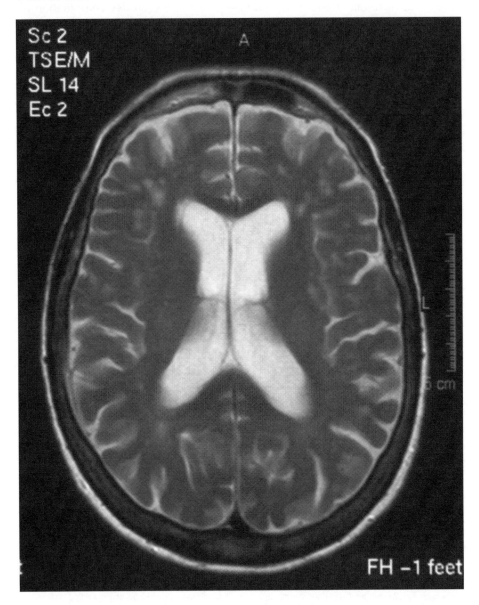

*Figure 5-III..A. MRI of the brain. This is a T2-weighted image, since the CSF spaces appear of high signal (white). Note the presence of several small areas of fluid density within the brain tissue, which are due to small areas of ischaemia.*

# MRCP (magnetic resonance colangiopancreatogram)

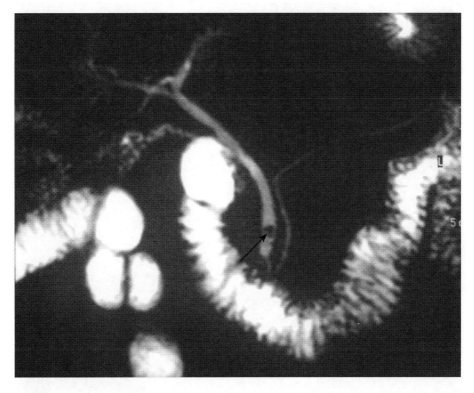

*Figure 5-III.B. MRCP showing a small filling defect within the distal common bile duct in keeping with a small calculus (arrow).*

# MRA (magnetic resonance angiogram)

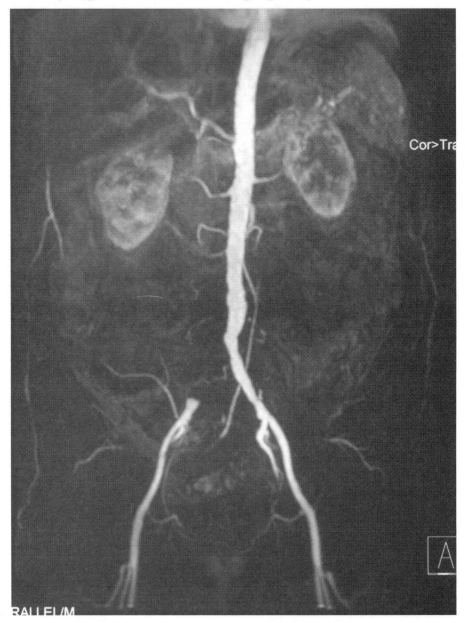

*Figure 5-III.C. MRA scan demonstrating the abdominal aorta, renal arteries, and iliac arteries. Note the occluded right common iliac artery.*

## MRI spine

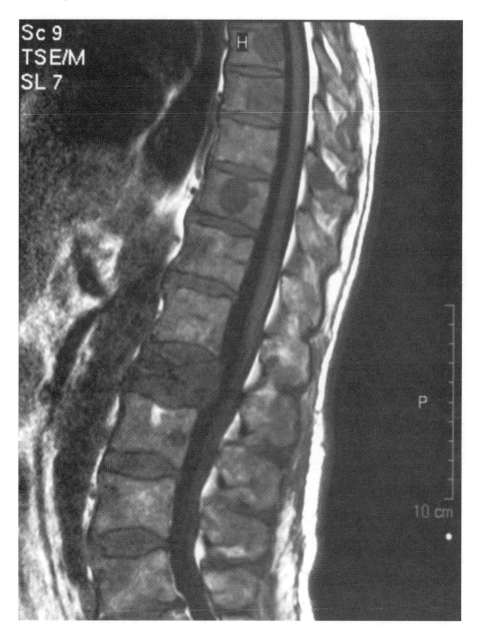

*Figure 5-III.D. MRI scan of the lumbar spine. This is a T1-weighted image (note the CSF is black cf. the appearances of Figure 5-III.A). There are multiple areas of low signal within several lumbar vertebral bodies. These are the appearances of diffuse metastatic deposits.*

# Section 6

# Computed Tomography
# of the Brain

# Introduction

Computed tomographic (CT) scanning of the brain has revolutionised the diagnosis and assessment of both neurological and neurosurgical cases over the last 20–30 years. More latterly, imaging of the brain and spine has been further aided by magnetic resonance imaging (MRI).

However, CT remains the radiological examination of choice in the evaluation of severe head injuries. CT clearly depicts acute intracranial haemorrhage, as well as demonstrating bone for associated fractures. In addition, CT scanning is widely available as an on-call service, and through the use of modern scanners, the scan times are short. Furthermore, as a distinction from MRI, there is no need for specialised anaesthetic equipment if an acutely ill patient should require ventilation or other supportive treatment at the time of scanning.

CT scanning of the brain does not require high-speed protocols because, unlike the thorax, the brain is not susceptible to movement artefact and the scans do not need to be performed on a single breath hold. Although more and more scanners are now of the spiral or multislice type, they are often programmed to perform simple axial-type images of the brain as described below.

For routine CT scanning of the brain, the scanner is set to provide 3–5-mm slices through the posterior fossa as far as the petrous temporal bones in order to avoid bone artefact. Above this level, 5-mm axial slices are performed. In view of the radiation dosage, the scanner gantry is usually angled in order to avoid repeated radiation exposure to the eyes.

Images can be manipulated after the scan has been performed in order to demonstrate either brain or soft tissue or to evaluate the bones of the cranial vault, which may be particularly important if there is a history of trauma. For further details of image processing see *Centering and window values in CT* (p. 180).

## Uses of CT scanning of the brain

In the acute clinical setting, CT is usually performed after acute severe head injury, in the evaluation of 'stroke' (to differentiate haemorrhagic from ischaemic causes) and in the acutely ill patient with focal neurological signs and impaired conscious level. CT may also be used to examine for focal intracranial abnormality due to malignancy or infection (abscess).

CT is also often performed in the initial work-up of a patient with likely meningitis, and particularly if there are focal neurological signs. However, in cases of non-complicated meningitis or encephalitis, the CT is usually normal and the diagnosis will depend upon lumbar puncture. It is imperative that performing a CT does not delay treatment or lumbar puncture.

CT is not the preferred initial investigation for suspected multiple sclerosis or acoustic neuroma. These pathologies are better diagnosed by MRI.

## The normal brain and fundamentals of CT interpretation

On an unenhanced CT scan of the brain (the so-called 'plain' scan) the normal grey/white matter differentiation can be appreciated because the myelin-containing white matter appears (paradoxically) as lower density (ie. darker) beneath the peripheral grey matter. Scan assessment relies on review of the CSF spaces for symmetry and the midline remaining central. The normal gyral–sulcal pattern should appear undistorted and symmetrical. There is often calcification in the choroid plexus and occasionally within the basal ganglia, and these appearances are especially common in the elderly. Other age-related changes should also be assessed, eg. the small size of the ventricular spaces in the paediatric and young adult age group, and the cortical atrophy and prominence of the CSF spaces common to octogenarians and beyond.

*Review of the scan is then primarily to differentiate haemorrhage or infarct from mass lesion (ie. intracerebral metastases or primary).*

*Acute haemorrhage* appears as high density (white) in the acute phase, but this slowly darkens to become iso-dense to brain tissue 7–10 days after the initial bleed. Darkening continues so that 2–3 weeks after the bleed the area is of lower density than brain tissue, and any associated mass effect is beginning to resolve.

In cases of cerebral *ischaemia* or *infarct* an immediate CT may be normal in the initial 6–12 hours. Occasionally, thrombus may be seen within the middle cerebral artery in the acute phase. This usually indicates that there will be significant subsequent developing infarction. As cerebral infarction becomes established, infarction is seen as low density (see *Table 6.1*). This may be adjacent to the ventricular spaces, suggesting ischaemia of diffuse deep white matter, or may be seen as focal areas (usually less than 1 cm in the basal ganglia) known as lacunar infarcts. Ultimately, if there is central vessel occlusion, this will result in low density of an entire vascular territory. Just as in acute haemorrhage, acute infarct often results in surrounding oedema in the acute phase.

**Table 6.1. Appearances of 'stroke' on CT (non-contrast enhanced)**

| Cause of 'stroke' | Appearance on CT | Nomenclature |
|---|---|---|
| Haemorrhage | White | High density |
| Infarct | Black | Low density |

Note that if intravenous contrast is given in cases of suspected infarction, then this may result in further problems of interpretation due to the apparently pathological luxury perfusion that develops adjacent to areas of ischaemia. In cases of clinical or radiographic uncertainty after initial plain scanning it is usually better to delay post-contrast scanning for 4–6 weeks until luxury perfusion is beginning to resolve. Indeed, repeat plain scanning at this time may then clearly demonstrate established and unequivocal infarct.

An abnormal *mass* will usually distort the normal gyral pattern, and may be associated with surrounding oedema. There will often be abnormal enhancement following the injection of intravenous contrast, which may also clarify subtle appearances on a pre-contrast scan.

---

**Key points of computed tomography of the brain**

- Appearances of 'stroke' on non-contrast-enhanced CT (see *Table 6.1*).
- Know from the following cases the appearances of subdural, extradural, subarachnoid and intracerebral haemorrhage.
- Understand the importance of patient age in CT brain interpretation.

---

## €ASE 6.1 Age-related cerebral atrophy

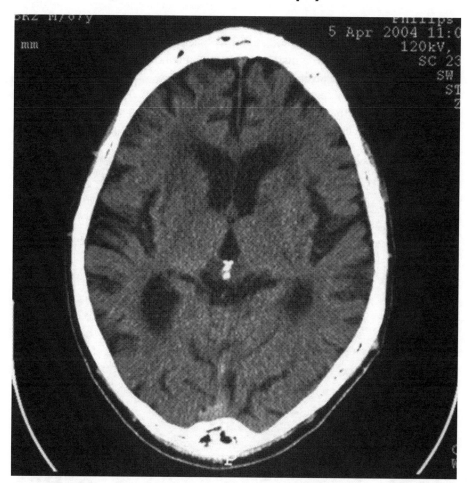

There is marked prominence of the sulci overlying the entire cerebral cortex. This patient was 85 years of age, and the appearances are in keeping with age-related atrophy. Note in addition, there is moderate periventricular (deep white matter) low density due to ischaemia in small-vessel disease. There is also a small focal area of lacunar infarction seen within the left basal ganglia, and thickening of the skull vault due to Paget's disease.

## Background

Cortical atrophy and prominence of the CSF spaces is common in octogenarians and beyond. There is usually associated CSF space dilation. Similar appearances can occur in patients with a history of chronic alcohol excess, which can also give marked cerebellar atrophy.

This age group of patients also often has evidence of deep white-matter ischaemia as is seen here, or small focal areas of infarction usually seen within the basal ganglia. These foci are known as lacunar infarcts (*Figure 6.1a*).

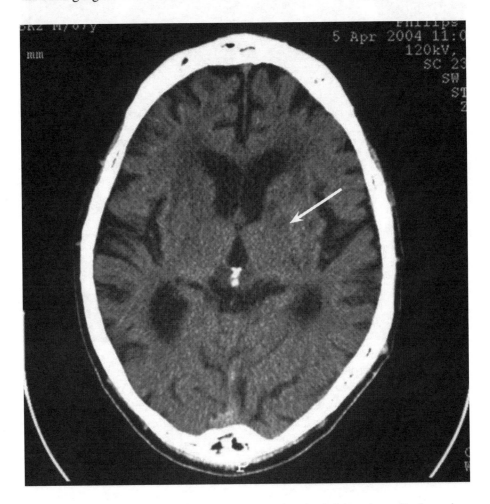

*Figure 6.1a. CT brain, showing lacunar infarct within the left basal ganglia (arrow).*

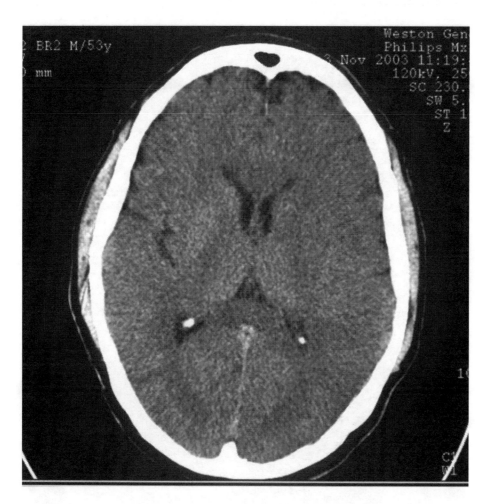

*Figure 6.1b. CT brain of a patient of approximately 25 years of age, with no evidence of significant atrophy, showing the ventricular system to be relatively slit-like in comparison with Figure 6.1a.*

Note the dramatic difference between the cases in *Figure 6.1a* and *Figure 6.1b*. The latter is the CT brain of a patient of approximately 25 years of age, with no evidence of significant atrophy.

## CASE 6.2 Subarachnoid haemorrhage

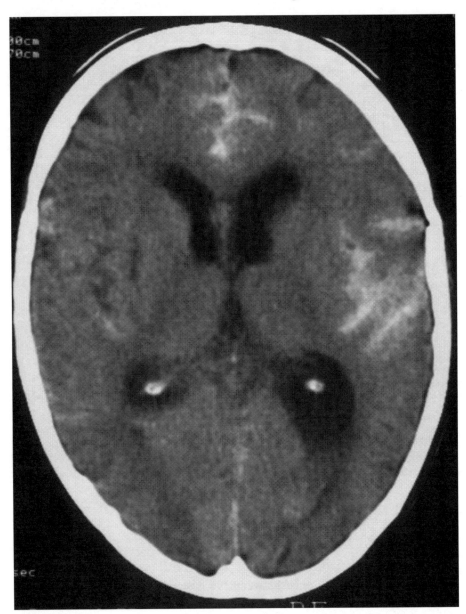

There is high density within the CSF spaces in keeping with acute subarachnoid haemorrhage. These appearances are most marked around the circle of Willis and into the left Sylvian fissure. They are likely to be due to ruptured left middle cerebral artery aneurysm.

## Background

Acute subarachnoid haemorrhage appears as high-density acute blood within the CSF spaces. This is often seen around the circle of Willis but can also extend over the cerebral hemispheres or into the Sylvian fissures. There may be evidence of secondary hydrocephalus due to the blood causing obstruction to the pacchionian corpuscles involved in CSF resorption. If there is a history of trauma, fractures may also be present.

The cause of a subarachnoid haemorrhage may also be indicated by the presence of an underlying aneurysm or arteriovenous malformation. These may demonstrate curvilinear calcification within their walls, but are best seen after the injection of intravenous contrast (*Figure 6.2a*). If the underlying causative lesion is not seen, the distribution of the subarachnoid blood may suggest the likely site of the underlying pathology. Ultimately, carotid angiography or (more latterly), MRA may be needed to reveal the underlying cause (see *Figure 5III.C*).

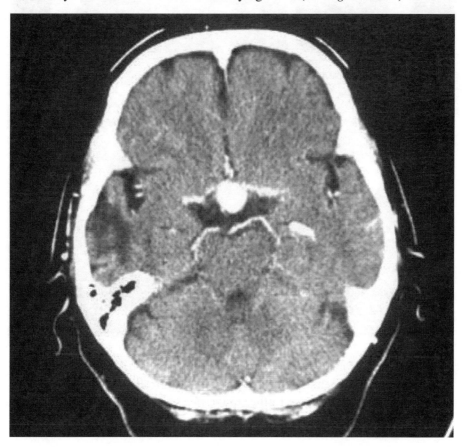

*Figure 6.2a. CT brain (post-IV contrast) showing enhancement of an anterior communicating artery aneurysm.*

## CASE 6.3 Intracerebral haematoma

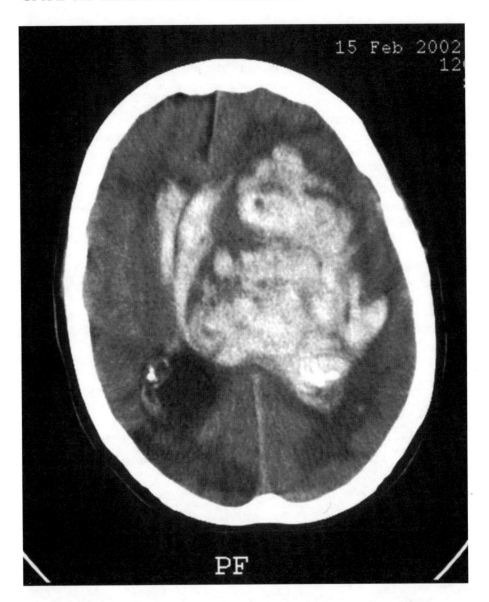

There is an area of increased density within the cerebral tissue, in keeping with acute intracerebral haematoma. There is marked surrounding low density due to oedema which contributes further to the mass effect and midline shift. The blood has also extended into the ventricular system.

## Background

An intracerebral haematoma appears as an area of increased density within the cerebral tissue. This is usually surrounded by low density (dark/black) due to peripheral oedema. Intracerebral haematomas often exert mass effect and result in compression of the adjacent CSF spaces. Blood may also extend into the ventricular system (*Figure 6.3a*). If there is a history of trauma, then a review on bone window settings may show an underlying fracture.

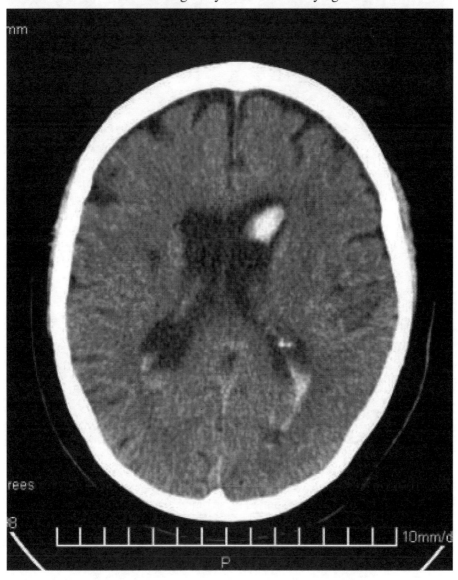

*Figure 6.3a. Acute blood, seen anteriorly in the left lateral ventricle, and as fluid levels within the posterior horns.*

## CASE 6.4 Acute extradural haematoma

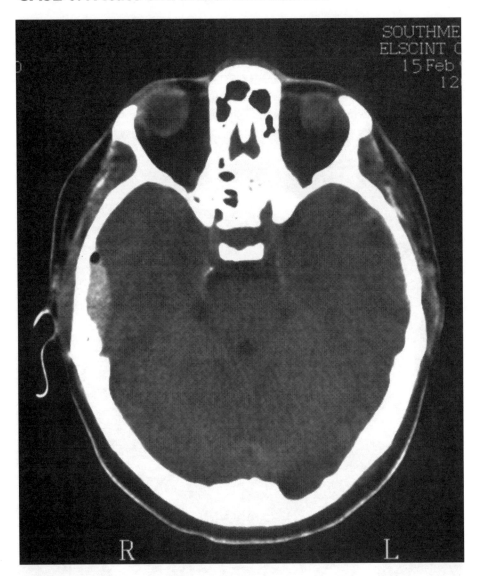

There is a lens-shaped (lentiform) area of high density overlying the right parietal lobe in keeping with acute extradural haematoma. A bubble of low density is also evident; this is due to intracranial gas and suggests that the dura has been breached.

## Background

A bleed in the extradural space presents as a lentiform (lens-shaped) peripheral area of high density. This forms as the collecting haematoma peels the dura from the inner table of the skull vault. The anatomical position of an extradural haematoma causes it to be limited by dural attachments and consequently these haematomas do not extend across suture lines. An underlying fracture of the skull vault may be seen, and occasionally intracranial gas may be seen if the dura has been breached. There may also be evidence of intracerebral contusion, manifested as a localised area of intracerebral high density (*Figure 6.4a*).

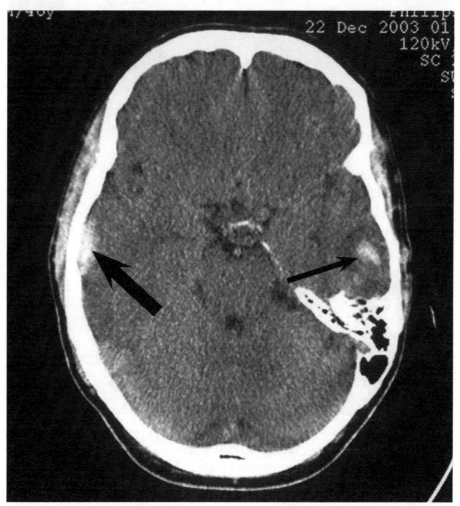

*Figure 6.4a. CT brain showing small right acute extradural haematoma (thick arrow), with associated left cerebral contusion (thin arrow).*

## CASE 6.5 Acute subdural haematoma

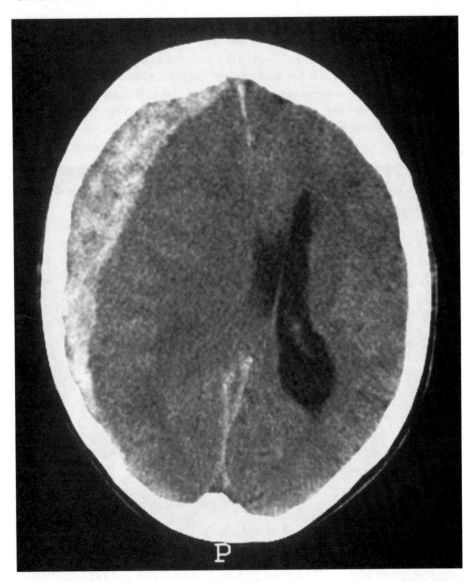

There is a peripheral area of high density overlying the right cerebral cortex, in keeping with acute subdural haemorrhage. There is severe associated mass effect, manifested by compression of the ventricular system and midline shift to the left side. The gyral–sulcal pattern is also part effaced for a patient of his age (in his 60s), suggesting raised intracranial pressure.

## Background

A bleed in the subdural space is seen as a peripherally located crescent of acute (high-density) blood. Bleeding into the subdural space is not limited by dural attachments at the sutures and the bleeding can therefore extend across the cerebral hemispheres. There may be significant mass effect (*Figure 6.5a*).

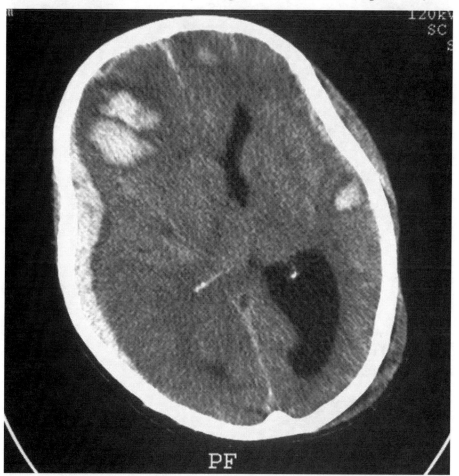

*Figure 6.5a. CT brain showing right acute subdural bleed, with significant mass effect. The areas of high density within the frontal lobes and on the left side of the patient are due to acute intracerebral haemorhage. There is developing hydrocephalus. Also note the subcutaneous occupital haematoma. All appearances are in keeping with significant trauma.*

## CASE 6.6 Chronic subdural haematoma

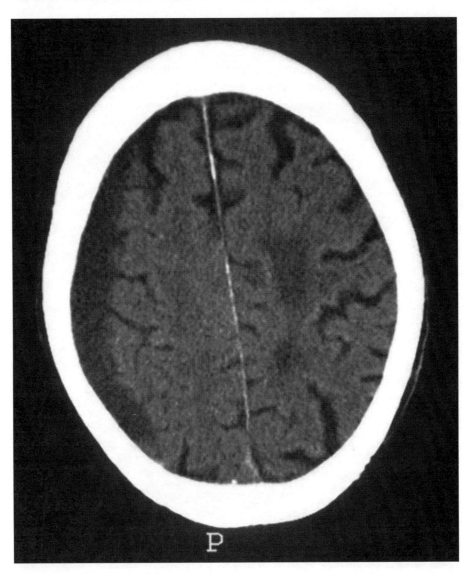

There is a peripheral area of low density overlying the left cerebral cortex, in keeping with chronic subdural haemorrhage. There is mild associated mass effect, with effacement of the sulcal pattern.

## Background

A chronic subdural haematoma demonstrates the same configuration as its acute counterpart, but it is of low density. There may be significant mass effect. Bilateral chronic subdural haematomas are occasionally seen and, although these result in a large amount of pressure effect, symmetry may be preserved, due to the pressures on each side counterbalancing one another (*Figure 6.6a*).

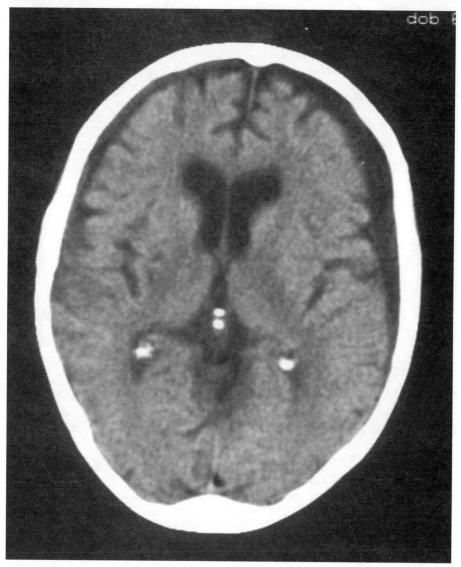

*Figure 6.6a. CT brain showing bilateral crescentic areas of low density in keeping with bilateral chronic subdural haematomas.*

## CASE 6.7 Ischaemia/infarct of right middle cerebral artery territory

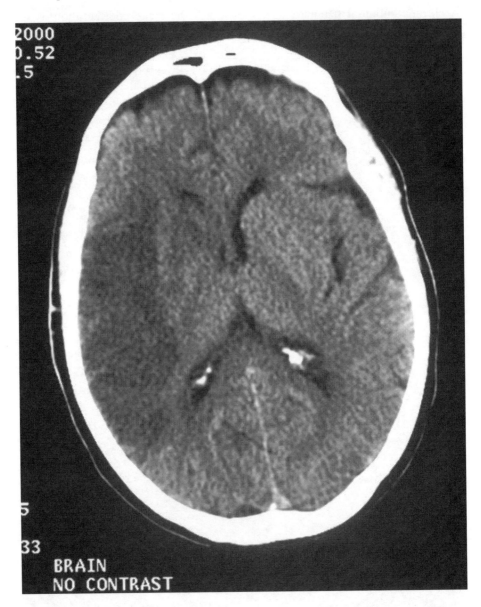

There is an area of low density within the right temporoparietal area. There is extension to the cortical surface, and there is loss of clear grey/white matter differentiation. There is some mass effect, with a little compression of the right lateral ventricle. The appearances are in keeping with acute right middle cerebral artery infarct.

## Background

A decrease in cerebral blood flow may result in cerebral ischaemia, and ultimately infarction. This usually occurs due to local thrombus or embolus. A CT scan performed within the initial 6–12 hours may be normal, but as cerebral infarction becomes established, low density develops in the vascular territory involved (*Figures 6.7a* and *6.7b*). Initially, there may be associated oedema and mass effect. There may be luxury perfusion in the periphery of the infarct, and small areas of haemorrhage may also be seen. With the passage of time, the oedema resolves, causing overall volume loss, and there may be resultant compensatory dilatation of the adjacent CSF spaces (*Figure 6.7c*).

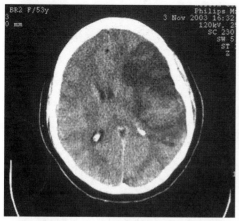

*Figure 6.7a. Acute middle cerebral artery infarct (note the mass effect due to acute ischaemic change and associated oedema).*

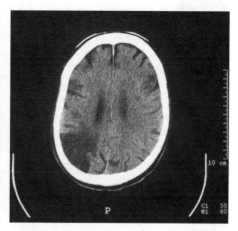

*Figure 6.7b. Posterior cerebral artery infarct.*

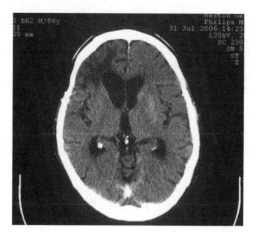

*Figure 6.7c. Longstanding infarct to right frontal cerebral artery territory with overall volume loss and ventricular expansion.*

## CASE 6.8 Intracerebral metastases

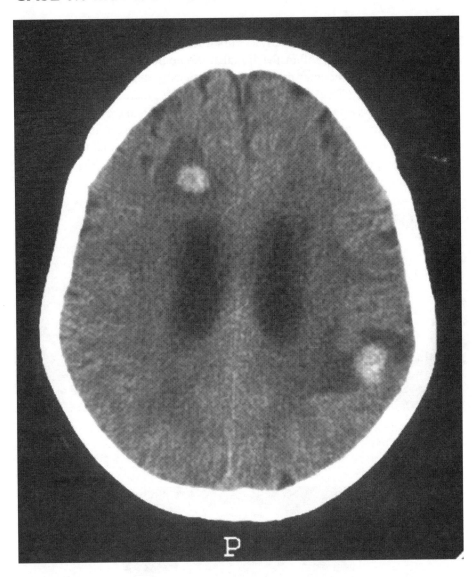

There are two areas of abnormal high density, primarily at the grey/white matter border. There is marked surrounding low density oedema. These appearances are in keeping with intracerebral metastases. This patient was known to have a history of malignant melanoma.

## Background

Metastases usually occur at the grey/white matter border and may be of increased or decreased density with respect to brain tissue. They are often multiple, and indeed their multiplicity is important for their radiographic diagnosis. Metastases usually induce marked surrrounding oedema, and usually enhance after contrast injection, either uniformly, or as a thick and irregular ring (*Figure 6.8a*). A history of previous malignancy is of importance in making the diagnosis. The most common tumours to metastasise to the brain are primary tumours of the bronchus, breast, kidney and stomach. Malignant melanoma shows the highest frequency of such secondary spread. Review of a recent CXR is often helpful to either demonstrate the primary lesion or to reveal further secondaries.

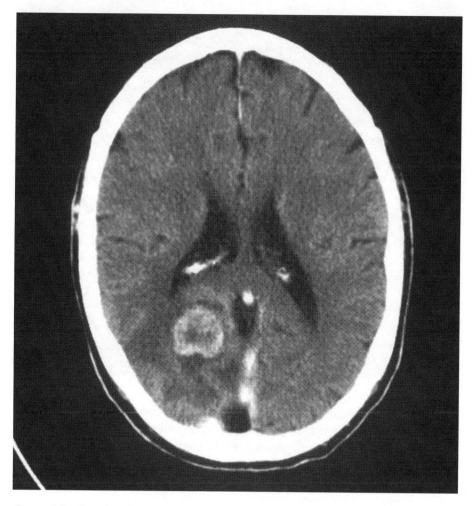

*Figure 6.8a. Peripherally enhancing metastasis in the right occipital lobe.*

## CASE 6.9 Astrocytoma

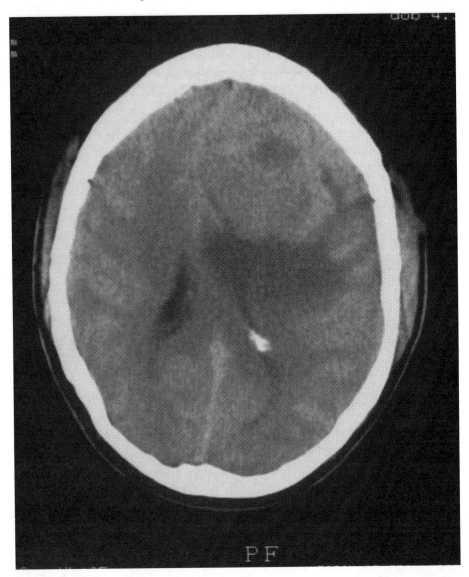

There is an area of low density within the left frontoparietal region, with mass effect and compression of the ventricular system. This is not typical of an acute bleed, and does not conform to a vascular territory. It is most likely to be due to an underlying mass lesion. On injection of intravenous contrast (in the next image) there is marked abnormal enhancement. The appearances are in keeping with primary malignancy; in view of the extent of the enhancement this is most likely due to malignant glioblastoma multiforme (aggressive astrocytoma).

## Background

These are the most common primary brain tumours in adults. They are graded from I to IV depending on their degree of malignancy. Radiologically, they appear as an intracranial mass lesion, often of low density or sometimes of mixed density, particularly if there has been a recent bleed into the tumour. There may be a severe oedema reaction adjacent to the mass, and this, in conjunction with the mass itself, can cause significant mass effect. Similarly, surrounding low density can occur due to local tumour invasion. There is usually a heterogeneous hypervascular enhancement pattern, the degree of which corresponds to the grade or aggressive nature of the tumour (*Figure 6.9a*). Calcification or cystic change can rarely occur at the more benign end of the pathological spectrum.

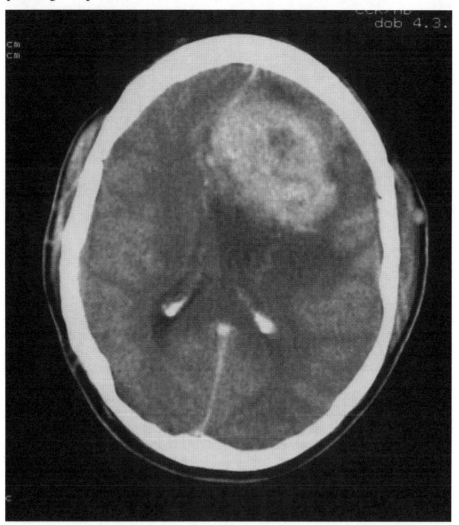

*Figure 6.9a. Repeated CT (same patient) with intravenous contrast, confirming pathological hypervascularity in keeping with aggressive primary malignancy.*

## CASE 6.10 Meningioma

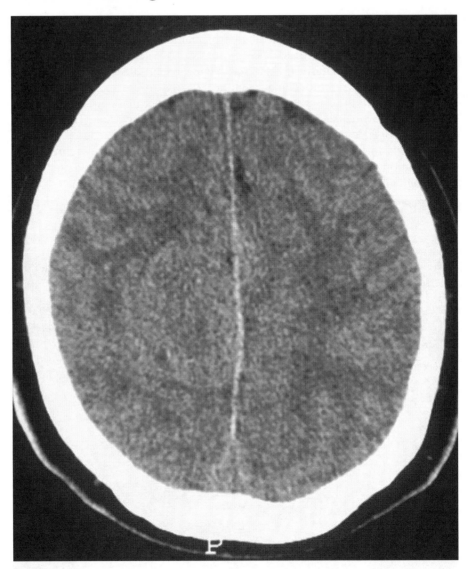

There is a smooth-edged, slightly hyperdense lesion arising from the inter-hemispheric fissure (falx). There is little surrounding oedema and there does not appear to be adjacent invasion. The appearances are in keeping with meningioma, and as shown on the right, this is concerned with the injection of intravenous contrast.

## Background

Meningiomas arise from the arachnoid granulations closely related to the venous sinuses, but they are also found over the convexity of the cerebral hemispheres. These tumours are 'extra-axial' in their position and thus compress rather than invade adjacent brain. Meningiomas are usually benign, although they can invade adjacent bone, or cause an adjacent osteosclerotic response. They are found anatomically in sites that correspond to their pathological origin, and thus they are commonly seen adjacent to the falx or sagittal sinus, over the convexity of the cerebral hemispheres, or at the skull base. Radiologically, meningiomas are usually uniformly hyperdense with respect to normal brain tissue and show dramatic, homogeneous enhancement after the injection of radiographic contrast medium (*Figure 6.10a*) – the 'light-bulb' sign. There may be a surrounding area of low density oedema in up to 20% of meningiomas, and uniform areas of calcification may also be present.

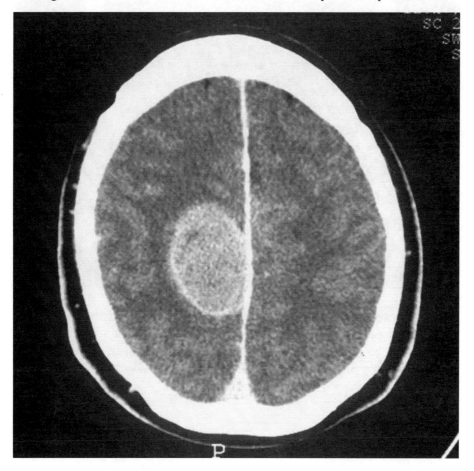

*Figure 6.10a. Repeated CT (same patient) with intravenous contrast, confirming uniform hypervascular enhancement in keeping with meningioma.*

## CASE 10.11 Intracerebral abscess

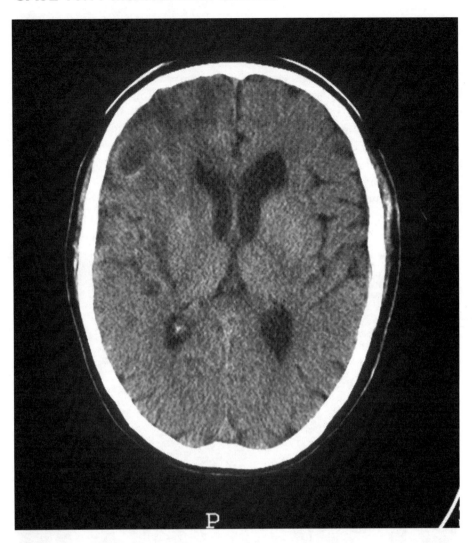

There are two areas of abnormal low density within the right frontal lobe, which show peripheral ring enhancement after the injection of intravenous contrast (see below). There is some surrounding low density oedema. These appearances are in keeping with intracerebral abscesses. This patient was known to be immunocompromised.

## Background

Intracerebral abscess must be suspected in a septic patient with neurological signs. Suspicion should be raised if there is a history of sinus disease, immunocompromise, intracardiac shunts, pulmonary abscess or subacute bacterial endocarditis. The radiological appearances may mimic those of an isolated metastasis, although the rim of enhancement is usually finer in outline, and while oedema is usually present, it is usually less marked. The adjacent sinuses should be evaluated for underlying infection. Although intracranial abscess is usually solitary, occasionally a daughter loculus is also present, as is seen here (*Figure 10.11a*). These abscesses were confirmed to be due to *Staphylococcus aureus*.

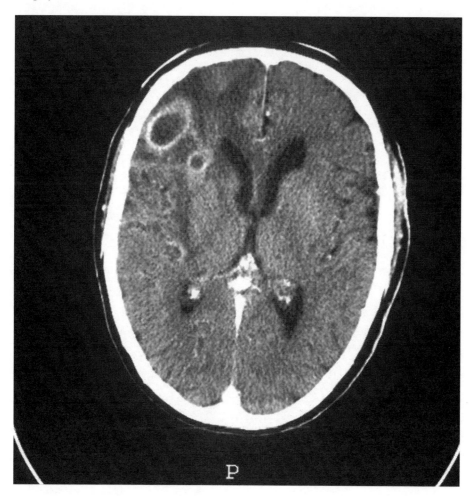

*Figure 10.11a. CT brain (same patient) after intravenous contrast, confirming a rim enhancement in right frontal lobe abscesses.*

# Section 7

# Interventional Radiology

## Introduction

The field of interventional radiology has expanded hugely in the last 20–30 years, due both to the development and refinement of small-calibre disposable equipment, and to the more varied and sophisticated collection of procedures possible. These procedures are minimally invasive to the patient, but may be technically challenging. To perform them safely requires close collaboration between the interventional radiologist and his or her clinical colleagues. Patients undergoing many of these procedures should be considered as though undergoing minimally invasive surgery.

Traditionally there has been a division of radiological intervention into arterial/vascular and non-vascular procedures.

### Vascular intervention

The mainstay of vascular intervention takes the form of angiography and angioplasty (see *Case 7.5*). In addition, a variety of embolisation techniques are used in the treatment of acute haemorrhage, or to decrease vascularity prior to surgery, or even in place of surgery (eg. uterine artery fibroid embolisation). Chemotherapy may also be given locally by, for example, passing a catheter into branches of the hepatic artery as close as possible to a known metastasis or previously diagnosed hepatocellular carcinoma. This allows a local high-concentration chemotherapy infusion to be given.

A variety of venous procedures may also be undertaken, including venous filters (see *Case 7.6*), venous stenting (usually of the superior vena cava compressed by metastatic disease to the mediastinum), or venous embolisation techniques (eg. testicular varicocoele embolisation).

### Non-vascular intervention

There is a wide range of potential non-vascular procedures possible, of which a small number are given in the case examples below.

These cases may involve intervention of the urinary tract, biliary tree, or gastrointestinal tract. The procedures are often preformed in order to palliate symptoms caused by inoperable malignancy, and they usually involve a minimally invasive approach (eg. percutaneous access being no more than 2–3 mm in length) and may allow the patient to be discharged home (or back to hospice care) within just a few days. In addition to such palliative procedures, a variety of biopsy and drainage techniques are also possible. Biopsy of an abdominal mass or lung lesion (*Case 7.4*) is common-place.

| | |
|---|---|
| **Key points of interventional radiology** | |

- Know the terms angiography, angioplasty and stent.
- Have an awareness of the range of non-vascular interventional procedures possible.
- If in doubt about the feasibility of a particular procedure, ask the advice of your local interventionalist.

## CASE 7.1 Oesophageal stenting

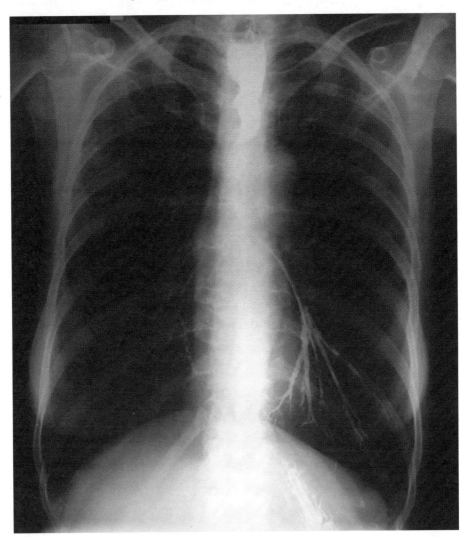

This chest radiograph was performed after a barium swallow examination. It confirms a stricture within the upper oesophagus, in keeping with an oesophageal carcinoma. In addition, barium has been aspirated into the bronchial tree on the left side. The patient should be referred to the physiotherapy department to help expectorate this. The tumour should be staged for the extent of spread. If it is irresectable, then oesophageal stenting may be appropriate.

This contrast swallow examination (different patient) shows a tight stricture in the lower oesophagus extending into the gastro-oesophageal junction. There is an irregular tail of contrast extending distally into the stomach. These are the appearances of a partially obstructing distal oesophageal carcinoma.

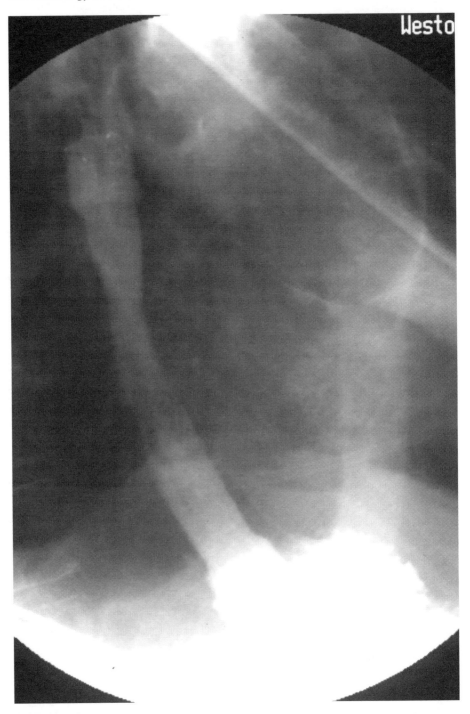

Westo

Radiological placement of an oesophageal stent is shown here. The area of the stricture is being distended by a recently deployed stent, and oral contrast is now beginning to pass into the stomach. A film at 24 hours will show further resolution of the strictured segment as the stent continues to expand.

## Background

A stent is a generic term for a prosthetic tube. The stent is usually inserted through the native tube (eg. bile duct, ureter, or as in this case the oesophagus) which has become obstructed and its placement will result in palliation of symptoms. Obstruction usually occurs due to malignancy where, due to the extent of the tumour involvement, a definitive operative resection is not possible. Stents are manufactured from plastic or metal, and their length and diameter will obviously correspond to the anatomical structure into which they are to be deployed.

Oesophageal stenting is an invaluable procedure in cases of severe or total dysphagia, due to inoperable carcinoma of the oesophagus.

Oesophageal stents are metallic and self-expanding (ie. are packaged in a collapsed form, and are released and allowed to expand when they have been positioned across the obstruction). They may have a plastic covering to impede tumour in-growth. They vary in their design, often having flared ends, or covered and uncovered parts that hold them in place across the obstructing tumour and thus prevent migration into the stomach. If a stent is deployed across the gastro-oesophageal junction, then gastro-oesophageal reflux can be severe and thus stents are available with an integral antireflux valve.

Stents may be inserted radiologically or endoscopically. Complications include blockage due to food bolus, aspiration, oesophageal perforation, pneumomediastinum, and migration (fall-through into stomach).

## CASE 7.2 Biliary stenting

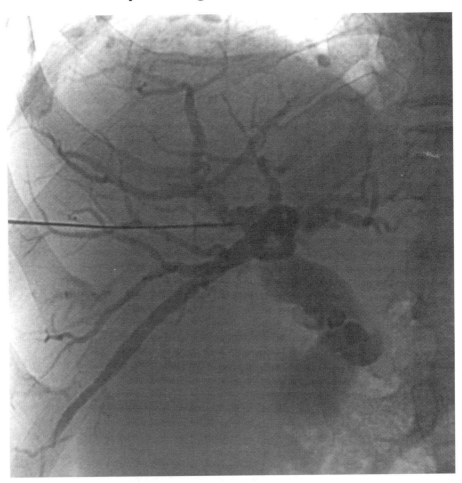

This is a percutaneous transhepatic cholangiogram (PTC). It demonstrates a tight stricture in the lower common bile duct, probably due to carcinoma of the pancreas. If the stricture is deemed inoperable on CT scanning and other staging criteria, then this procedure will allow the subsequent deployment of a metallic biliary stent. This will allow the biliary system to drain internally into the duodenum, and help resolve the obstructive jaundice and its associated symptoms.

## Background

Biliary stents are usually placed for inoperable carcinomas of the pancreas or cholangiocarcinomas of the bile ducts, which are causing obstructive jaundice. They are often placed endoscopically at ERCP (endoscopic retrograde cholangiopancreatography), but if the patient has had previous gastric surgery or the tumour is large the papilla within the duodenum may not be accessible or visible. The stent is therefore deployed percutaneously. This is performed under ultrasound and

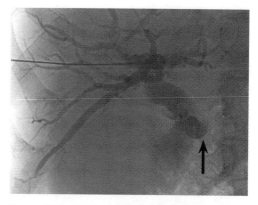

Figure 7.2a. PTC in the same case demonstrating stricture in the lower common bile duct (arrow).

fluoroscopic (X-ray screening) guidance, first by achieving access into the biliary tree by PTC and then crossing the stricture to place the self-expanding metal stent. The stent will allow drainage into the duodenum (*Figures 7.2a and 7.2b*). An external biliary drain is often left in situ temporarily should the stent become blocked, and to allow the system to fully decompress. Complications of this procedure include internal bleeding, cholangiitis and biliary peritonitis.

Prior to any hepatic intervention (eg. liver biopsy) normal blood clotting and platelet levels should be confirmed. Antibiotic cover should also be given prior to PTC or biliary stenting. The patient should have undergone fully informed written consent, as with any interventional procedure.

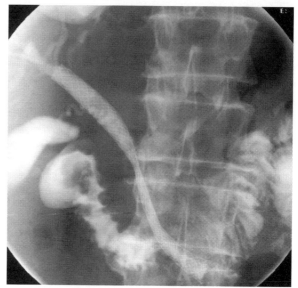

Figure 7.2b. A metallic biliary stent has now been placed across the biliary stricture and contrast can be seen to flow into the duodenum.

## CASE 7.3 Uretic stenting

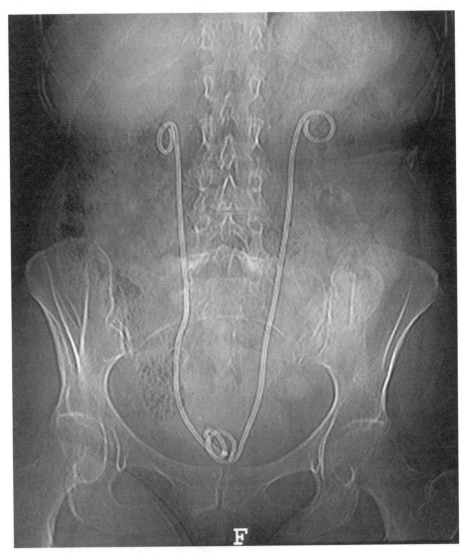

This is a so-called 'scout' film, or topogram, which is performed in the planning of a CT scan. It shows bilateral double 'J' ureteric stents (so called because of the J-shaped loops at each end) positioned satisfactorily between the renal pelvis and the urinary bladder.

## Background

Patients with obstructive renal failure due to large inoperable pelvic tumours may be treated palliatively by insertion of a nephrostomy. A nephrostomy is a drain in the renal collecting system, which is usually inserted under ultrasound and fluoroscopic guidance. This allows an obstructed kidney to drain externally. The patient is often given light sedation and antibiotics prior to the procedure. Following this procedure a ureteric stent may be deployed antegradely (ie. passed down the ureter from the kidney into the bladder) to allow internal drainage to the bladder. The nephrostomy tube may then be removed. In the case example, the stents are seen to be lying within the ureters, which are both medially positioned. This is because this patient is suffering from retroperitoneal fibrosis, that is fibrosis within the retroperitoneal tissues which has caused bilateral ureteric obstruction and traction towards the midline. In this case, it was due to the patient taking the drug methysergide.

The complications that can follow urological interventional procedures include infection and bleeding, although thrombus within the collecting system is usually rapidly broken down by urinary urokinase.

Stents may of course also be passed retrogradely (from the bladder back up into the kidney). This procedure is undertaken by a urologist in theatre.

Other causes of retroperitoneal fibrosis include:

- Retroperitoneal malignancy (lymphoma or metastases from breast/colon carcinoma) due to the tumour initiating a fibrotic reaction.
- Inflammatory conditions (eg. diverticular disease or Crohn's disease).
- Aortic aneurysm.
- Trauma.
- Surgery.
- Drugs (eg. methysergide).
- Idiopathic (actually more than 50% of cases).

## CASE 7.4 CT-guided lung biopsy

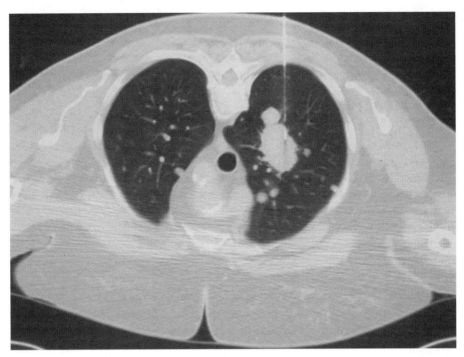

This is a single image from a CT-guided lung biopsy. CT-guided lung biopsies are classically used to determine histology of peripheral lung mass, that is a mass which is close to or abutting the pleural surface. However, the biopsy of more central lung parenchymal lesions is possible if histology cannot be gained from bronchoscopy or from sputum cytology.

## Background

The potential risks of this procedure include the following:

- pneumothorax
- haemoptysis
- haemorrhage
- pain.

Historically, the incidence of pneumothorax is said to be 10%, when determined by chest X-ray. However the biopsy of smaller more central lesions and the evaluation by CT instead of plain radiography have shown that pneumothorax can occur in as many as 60% of cases, although the majority of these do not require active management.

Reassessment of these patients is necessary after the biopsy to determine whether pneumothorax has occurred. This is often done with a limited CT immediately post-biopsy procedure (see *Figure 7.4a*), and by a CXR at 2 hours post-biopsy.

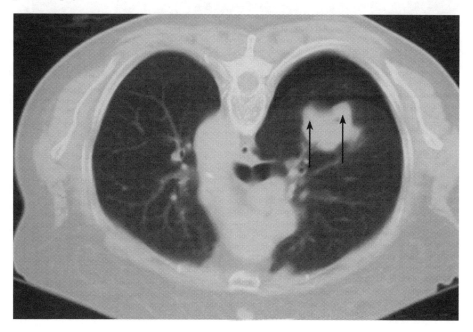

*Figure 7.4a. CT chest post lung biopsy showing small pneumothorax (arrows).*

The use of CT allows biopsy of deeper smaller lesions than was previously possible. *Figure 7.4b,* for example, is a case of para-aortic lymph node biopsy.

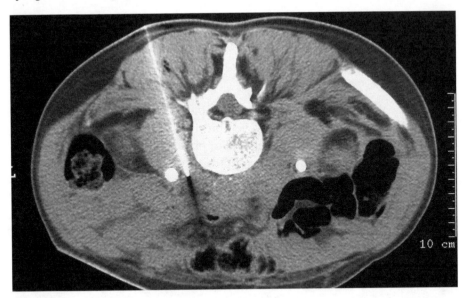

Figure 7.4b. CT abdomen (with patient prone) showing needle track into para-aortic lymph node. This biopsy confirmed a diagnosis of lymphoma. The high density adjacent to the needle tip is contrast within the ureter. The contrast was administered before the biopsy to allow visualisation of the ureter, so it could be avoided when the needle was passed. .

## CASE 7.5 Angiography/angioplasty

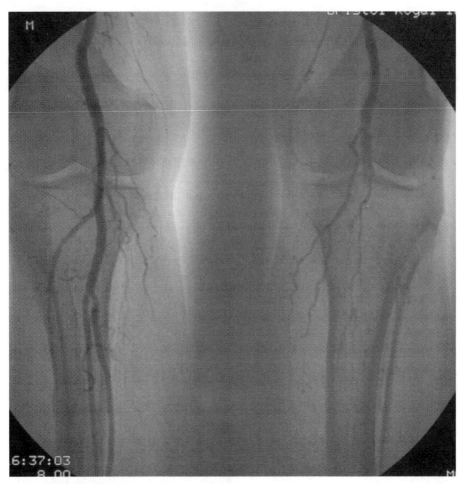

This is a digital subtraction angiogram (DSA) of the popliteal arteries. It demonstrates an abrupt 'cut-off' of contrast within the left popliteal artery. The abrupt nature of the obstruction and the absence of extensive collateral arteries or of adjacent atherosclerotic disease, suggests this is most likely to be due to embolus, rather than chronic arterial disease. This patient was found to be in atrial fibrillation which is a major risk factor for the development of peripheral emboli. Emboli such as this require surgical removal. Post surgery, an echocardiogram of the heart should be performed to exclude a source for embolic material and to assess cardiac function. These patients should usually be anticoagulated with warfarin.

## Background

DSA allows a 'road map' of images of the arterial anatomy to be obtained, which will show evidence of atherosclerotic stenoses or occlusions, and is invaluable for diagnostic purposes. It is performed prior to angioplasty (ballooning) (see *Figures 7.5a–c*) or arterial stenting (a metallic tube to hold a heavily diseased artery open). Angiography can be performed of any body region, but DSA is of particular use within the legs, and coronary and cerebral circulations.

The technique involves introducing a catheter (a fine plastic tube) through which intra-arterial contrast can be injected. The majority of cases are performed by introducing the catheter through a tiny incision of 1–2 mm in the femoral artery. A digital film is initially taken of each area. Arterial contrast is then injected and further films are taken. The initial film is then digitally subtracted from these films, to leave a final image that only shows arterial contrast.

Although angiography is widely used and allows arterial intervention in the form of angioplasty, other non-invasive investigative techniques including duplex ultrasound, CT, and MR angiography (see *Case 5-III.C*) are being used increasingly to assess peripheral vessels.

The main complications of angiography include haematoma at the puncture site within the femoral artery and, less commonly, thrombus or embolus due to the passage of catheters or wires through heavily diseased vessels. These risks are of course avoided by the non-invasive imaging techniques.

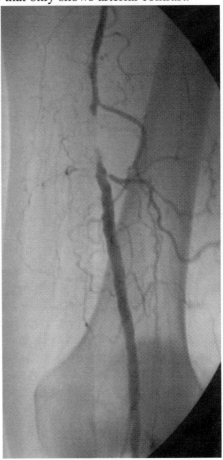

Figure 7.5a. Digital subtraction angiogram showing short occlusion within the distal left superficial femoral artery.

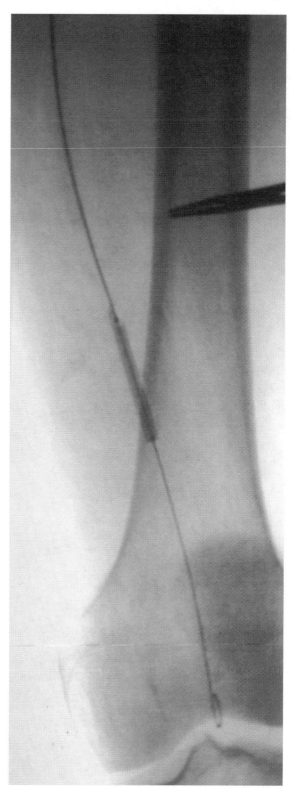

Figure 7.5b. Film showing an angiography wire crossing the occluded segment, and an angioplasty balloon positioned within the occlusion (radio-opaque markers are present at each end of the balloon).

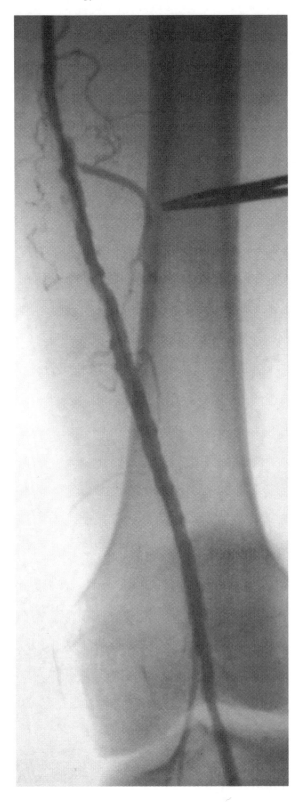

Figure 7.5c. Post-angioplasty digital subtraction angiogram after the balloon has been deflated and removed, showing reperfusion through the previously occluded segment.

## CASE 7.6 Inferior vena cava (IVC) filters

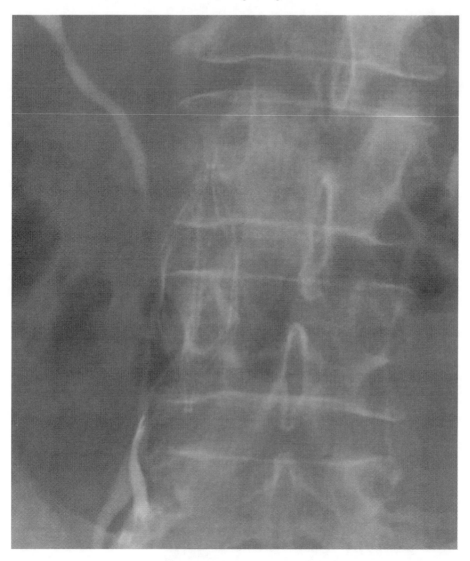

This is a localised magnified view of the central abdomen showing a filter device within the inferior vena cava (IVC).

## Background

IVC filters are inserted under fluoroscopic control, via either the femoral or jugular veins. They are positioned as seen here in the lower IVC below, the level of the renal veins (*Figure 7.6a*). IVC filters are designed to capture thrombi passing from the deep veins of the legs, and in so doing will prevent pulmonary emboli in more than 90% of cases. They are used according to the following criteria:

- In patients with confirmed thromboembolic disease (deep vein thrombosis or pulmonary embolus) who under ordinary circumstances would be anticoagulated, but due to concomitant pathology (eg. haemorrhagic stroke or gastrointestinal bleed) cannot be anticoagulated in the normal way.
- In patients who are already appropriately anticoagulated for thromboembolic disease, but are still developing pulmonary emboli.
- In patients known to be of high risk of thromboembolic disease who are then undergoing pelvic surgery, thus increasing their risk still further. The filters used in these cases are usually temporary, and can be removed when the additional risk factors have passed. Similarly, patients who have experienced severe trauma may be given temporary filters in some centres.

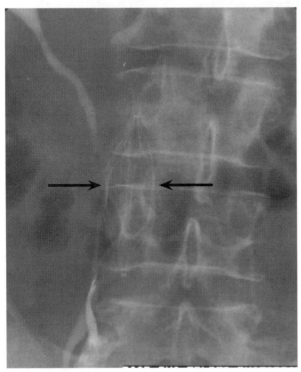

*Figure 7.6a. Magnified view of the filter device (arrows) in the same patient. .*

# Index